Midwest Mediterranean 2.0

Finding Health & Flavor with the Foods of the North

THERAN PRESS

THERAN PRESS IS THE ACADEMIC PUBLISHING IMPRINT OF SILVER GOAT MEDIA.

THERAN IS DEDICATED TO AUTHENTIC PARTNERSHIPS WITH OUR ACADEMIC ASSOCIATES, TO THE QUALITY DESIGN OF SCHOLARLY BOOKS, AND TO ELITE STANDARDS OF PEER REVIEW.

THERAN SEEKS TO FREE INTELLECTUALS FROM THE CONFINES OF TRADITIONAL PUBLISHING.

THERAN SCHOLARS ARE AUTHORITIES AND REVOLUTIONARIES IN THEIR RESPECTIVE FIELDS.

THERAN ENCOURAGES NEW MODELS FOR GENERATING AND DISTRIBUTING KNOWLEDGE.

FOR OUR CREATIVES, FOR OUR COMMUNITIES, FOR OUR WORLD.

WWW.THERANPRESS.ORG

SGM

This book was designed and produced by Silver Goat Media, LLC. Fargo, ND U.S.A.
www.silvergoatmedia.com

SGM, the SGM goat, Theran Press, and the Theran theta are trademarks of Silver Goat Media, LLC.

Cover design and typeset by Jonathan Rutter © 2025 SGM

ISBN-13: 978-1-944296-34-6

Jeremiah Program | FARGO MOORHEAD

A portion of the annual proceeds from the sale of this book is donated to the Jeremiah Program, Fargo-Moorhead. **www.jeremiahprogram.org**

Midwest Mediterranean 2.0

Finding Health & Flavor with the Foods of the North

Sean Ballinger, Susan Mathison, Megan Myrdal,
Brynn Peterson, Mark Rostad, Peter Schultz & Shelby Terstriep

Theran Press

For our friends, families, farmers, and fellow food lovers
—from the Midwest to the Mediterranean—
and everywhere in between.

CONTENTS

CONTRIBUTORS

Sean Ballinger (BA, Minnesota State University Moorhead) is an amateur philosopher, scholar, and scientist. His scientific interests are diverse, encompassing topics from grape breeding to the nature of religious experience. Professionally, he's dedicated to Bear Creek Winery in Fargo, ND, where he serves as the winemaker, vineyard manager, and head of research.

Susan Mathison (BA, Stanford University; MD, University of Texas, Southwestern, Dallas) is a mother, physician, surgeon, entrepreneur, volunteer, writer, and former farm wife. In 2002, she founded Catalyst Medical Center + Clinical Spa in Fargo, ND, to help her patients lead happier, healthier, and more beautiful lives. She has donated land and resources to support Growing Together Community Gardens and Farm in the Dell of the Red River Valley. She treasures time with her son, Grant; her mom, Marge; and her six siblings and their kids. She has served on numerous philanthropic and corporate boards; Dakota Medical Foundation, Impact Foundation, and Fargo Moorhead Science Museum hold special places in her heart. She serves as a health consultant for a wellness retreat in Santorini, Greece, and now carries Mediterranean sunshine in her Scandinavian heart.

Megan Myrdal (MS, North Dakota State University; RD, Concordia College) is a wife, mother, registered dietitian, farmer's daughter, and a general enthusiast for all things farming and food. She's a Senior Director of Development with the NDSU Foundation and a co-founder of both Food of the North and the Little Free Garden project. Her work experiences have spanned the food and agriculture industries, including nutrition and culinary education, food system policy, farmers market development, agriculture marketing, and higher learning. Throughout her career, Megan has learned that the people who care deeply about food are some of the best folks on the planet; supporting this community is the source of her daily motivation. She resides in Thompson, ND, with her family.

Brynn Peterson (BA, Concordia College; OD, Pacific University College of Optometry) is an art enthusiast, gardener, optometrist, and lifelong learner. She's lived in a variety of places—from the Pacific Northwest to the Driftless Area in western Wisconsin—and during her adventures has developed an interest in regional agriculture and food that she brought back to her own garden. This interest in nutrition and local food dovetails with her optometry practice as lifestyle choices make a significant impact in overall health and well-being. She practices primary care optometry at Eyecare Associates in Fargo, ND, with special interests in ocular disease and the role of systemic health in ocular disease.

Mark Rostad (BA, Concordia College; MD, North Dakota School of Medicine) grew up in Kindred, ND. He completed his residency in internal medicine at Gundersen Health System in La Crosse, WI. Chosen to serve as chief resident for a year after finishing residency, Mark went on to complete a fellowship in hospice and palliative medicine at the University of Iowa. After his training, he and his wife, Brynn, moved back home to North Dakota with their daughter, Ingrid, to be closer to family. In doing so, Mark became only the fourth fellowship-trained palliative care and hospice physician in the state of North Dakota. He began his medical practice as the inpatient palliative care physician at Essentia Health in Fargo, ND. In 2025, after four years at Essentia, Mark left and joined Hospice of the Red River Valley, where he currently serves as medical director.

Peter Schultz (BA, Concordia College; MA, Vanderbilt University; PhD, University of Athens) is an archaeologist, entrepreneur, and conservationist. He was the founding director of the Longspur Prairie Fund and is the principal and owner of Aegean Imports, LLC. Peter has held advanced fellowships from the Fulbright Foundation, the National Endowment for the Humanities, the A.G. Leventis Foundation, the American School of Classical Studies, among many others. His interests include ancient Greek art and literature, regenerative agriculture, the philosophy of mind, and global education. His most recent academic books are *The Thymele at Epidauros. Healing, Space, and Musical Performance in Late Classical Greece* (Theran Press, 2017), *Artists and Artistic Production in Ancient Greece* (Cambridge University Press, 2017), and *Speaking the Past. Heritage, Discourse, and Publishing in the Digital Age* (Theran Press, 2021).

Shelby Terstriep (BA & MD, University of Missouri–Kansas City) is a wife, mother, and medical oncologist/hematologist. She was a resident and fellow at the Mayo Clinic and serves as the medical director of Sanford Health's Cancer Survivorship Program. Passionate about helping cancer survivors thrive, Shelby focuses on minimizing the long-term effects of cancer and its treatment while empowering people to live healthier lives. Beyond medicine, Shelby's love for cooking and entertaining inspired her to co-found 701 Eateries, Brewbird, and City Brew Hall, where she brings people together over great food and warm hospitality.

ACKNOWLEDGMENTS

First, we collectively acknowledge that, here in the Midwest, we live and eat from the traditional lands of the Nu'eta (Mandan), Hidatsa, Sanish (Arikara), Lakota/Dakota, and Anishinabe/Ojibwe/Chippewa people. If you live in Minnesota, then you may live on lands that were of the eleven American Indian tribes that have borders within the state. It is through the removal, relocation, forced assimilation, unkept treaty obligations, and other policies of the United States and state governments that the health and lives of Indigenous people have been damaged. It is Indigenous people who experience some of the highest rates of food insecurity throughout the Midwest. With this in mind, let us work together in a just way to acknowledge and repair what we can of this harm. Let us also acknowledge the resilience and creativity of people working in food and agriculture, and work toward true justice in land and food access. Let us respect and learn from Indigenous people who have always recognized the true connections between a healthy Earth, healthy lands, and healthy people.

Additionally, Susan Mathison would like to thank her parents for their generous support and love; her siblings for their humor and connection; her son, Grant, for expanding her heart and mind beyond measure; and her Catalyst colleagues for living our mission to help others lead happier, healthier, more beautiful lives. Megan Myrdal would like to thank her grandmother Rosemarie for inspiring her love of food and farming; her sister Kierstin for the thoughtful edits and guidance on her chapter; and Kade, Haakon, Leif, and Harry for being her guinea pigs in all her Midwest Mediterranean culinary trials and errors. Peter Schultz would like to express his gratitude to his American family (Roger, Ruth, Liz, Eric, Anna, Dave, William, and Darcie) and to his Greek family (Eugene, Olga, Giannis, and Ero) for their endless kindness; in many ways, this project is theirs, too. Shelby Terstriep would like to thank her husband, Chad, and her kids, Elise, Drew, and Lauren, for their love and support! Finally, the publication of this book would not have been possible without the support of the Theran Press and its advisory board; the authors are happy to thank the press for its generosity, positivity, and good humor.

IMPORTANT NOTE. The information in this book is not a substitute for professional medical advice on specific physical or mental disorders or other physiological or emotional concerns. Please carefully consult with your doctor before changing, stopping, or starting any new diet, treatment, or medication.

Food for us comes from our relatives, whether they have wings or fins or roots. That is how we consider food. Food has a culture. It has a history. It has a story. It has relationships.

—Winona LaDuke

Let food be thy medicine and medicine be thy food.

—Hippocrates

People who aren't interested in food always seem rather dry and unloving—they just don't seem to have a real gusto for life.

—Julia Child

Introduction
Mediterranean Eating in the American Midwest . . . 2.0!

Megan Myrdal and Peter Schultz

So, here we are talking about a *Mediterranean*-style diet that's grounded in the upper *Midwest*—again!

And, once again, you might be asking—*why*?

Why are we still talking about food from areas like Italy, Turkey, Lebanon, North Africa, and Greece up here in the High Plains of North America? Why are we still looking at the food from places thousands of miles from home, from places with climates, cultures, landscapes, and cuisines that—at first glance—are so dramatically different from our own?

In other words, why are we still looking way over *there* to learn how to eat right *here*?

Well, there are several important reasons that you'll read about in this book, but first there's our origin story, a story centered around exceptionally delicious extra-virgin olive oil.

In 1997, Peter began his PhD in Greece. There, he met Eugene Ladopoulos, a Greek farmer and olive oil producer, and discovered Mr. Ladopoulos's "liquid gold"—the famous and wildly popular Mistra Estates extra-virgin olive oil. At that time, Mr. Ladopoulos's family had owned land and olive trees near ancient Sparta for generations, but that year was his first attempt to sell his oil in the US. Peter was astonished by the flavor and quality of this oil, and was impressed with the exceptional care Eugene took of his trees and his lands. Over time, Peter joined Eugene on his mission to bring this liquid gold to America—founding Peter Schultz, Importer (www.peterschultzimporter.com) and delivering this world-class product to friends and families across the upper Midwest.

Fast forward to 2019.

We were working together on a number of projects centered on "cultivating sustainable habits"—a phrase that Megan often uses to describe our work—and Peter asked Megan if she'd be interested in creating a recipe using Mistra Estates extra-virgin olive oil that featured locally grown, Midwest ingredients. Megan agreed and created the (now-famous) Midwest Mediterranean Bean Salad, which you can find in *Midwest Mediterranean* 1.0 on pages 61–62. This salad was a clean, simple dish featuring seasonal kale, cucumbers, tomatoes, onions, and herbs from our local Red River Market as well as dry edible beans that are grown in abundance across the upper Midwest, all paired with classic Mediterranean ingredients—balsamic vinegar, feta cheese, olives, and extra-virgin olive oil. It wasn't a complicated, fancy, or high-end recipe—it was simple home cooking! And it was freaking *delicious*! Indeed, everyone who's tasted this little salad has been blown away by how incredible *Midwest*-grown ingredients can taste when paired with key flavors of the *Mediterranean*. We knew that we had something there and that "something" was an idea, namely the idea that local, healthy Midwest-grown ingredients could be brilliantly paired with the techniques, foods, and recipes of the Mediterranean for both flavor and health. We both saw it. We both *tasted* it! There was something happening, and it was truly magical!

And, just like that, *Midwest Mediterranean* was born.

Now, we both knew that Megan could speak with knowledge on dietary issues, and that Peter could talk about olive oil for days on end.

But that wasn't enough.

To continue to feed the flames of this idea, to continue to crystallize our message, we realized that we needed a wider range of experts. This kind of project wasn't just about nutrition or ingredients or history, it was also about human biology, local ecologies, fair agriculture, deep sustainability, a passion for truly great living—and so much more! We were enthusiastic, but we clearly needed to add more experts to the team.

Over the next several months, we asked a number of brilliant advocates and physicians for this way of eating and living to join our journey and—*Voila!*—the first volume of *Midwest Mediterranean. Finding Health and Flavor with the Foods of the North* was born! (You can find this book on Amazon or anywhere high quality books are sold.) What made this so exciting was not just the great food but also the spirit of authentic community collaboration that guided every aspect of that little book's composition. And—maybe most importantly—we had a blast! To make a long story short, that first book—and its associated meals and events and mojo—was such a success that we decided we had to do it again.

And that brings us to this present volume.

The book that you hold now in your hands follows the exact template of *Midwest Mediterranean* 1.0. The difference is in the subjects of the chapters and the specifics of the sample recipes. Our themes are the same: to explore and celebrate the beneficial fusion of Mediterranean and Midwestern cuisines. Our goals are the same, too: to live and to eat extraordinarily well. But the areas of research and the examples of flavors are entirely different. This time, for example, instead of a brilliant cardiologist (David Clardy) talking about the benefits of the Mediterranean diet for heart health, we have a brilliant oncologist (Shelby Terstriep) talking about the importance of the Mediterranean diet as part of an anti-cancer regime. Instead of a local farmer dedicated to the production of healthy, high-quality ingredients (Noreen Thomas), we have a local oenologist (Sean Ballinger) dedicated to the production of delicious, high-quality wine. You get the idea. The principles of the first book work. So why not do more? Why not share more? Why not continue to bring these two communities and cultures together for more bounty, more health, more happiness?

Indeed, to close this introduction, it might be worthwhile to reflect a moment on this notion of what our little Midwest Mediterranean *community* has meant to us. Both our books were written by teams of Midwesterners from diverse backgrounds, a team of members that share a zeal for healthy food, healthy lives, and healthy souls. Both our books dip into history, agriculture, biology, philosophy, botany, ingredients, lifestyle, and more. Both our books are packed with a collection of amazing Midwest Mediterranean recipes created by, yet again, even more community collaborators: chefs and home cooks from across the Midwest and the Mediterranean who are truly passionate about this diet and this way of life. Our point is that this little book you now hold in your hands isn't just a "cookbook." It's not just a "health book" or a "diet book," either. And it's certainly not just a "book about food." Even more so than last time, we can say that this project is truly an amazing smorgasbord of principles and particulars—a kind of eclectic community table that we've all helped create for each other, a table at which we can all sit, share, learn, and enjoy. In this case, once again, the table is loaded with some truly life-changing ideas that we feel deserve the widest possible audience. In that spirit, we're honored to offer this book to the community that gave it life, with the hopes that we can all continue to enjoy learning and thinking about the food, the people, the recipes, and the stories that connect us to this amazing way of eating and living.

Chapter One
A Brief History of the Siesta

Peter Schultz, PhD

The people who cook and eat around the Mediterranean Sea cook and eat a wide variety of food. And yet, despite this variety, Mediterranean cuisine shares many common nutritional characteristics. If you've read the first volume of *Midwest Mediterranean*, then you've already been initiated into many of this diet's mysteries. If you haven't read *MWM* 1.0, then you're going to learn a ton about this diet's benefits in the next six chapters of this book. Right here in chapter 1, however, I don't want to talk about food. Rather, I'd like to share with you the many benefits of one of the Mediterranean diet's most well-known, most misunderstood, and most glorious traditions: The afternoon nap, also known as . . . *drumroll* . . . the siesta!

So, why talk about midday snoozing in a book about "diet?"

In ancient Greek, the word for "diet" is δῐαιτᾰ. The ancient word changes only slightly in modern Greek–to δίαιτα. This word is transliterated *díaita* and pronounced with the stress on the first syllable, like this: DEE-ai-ta. In both ancient and modern usage, the Greek word *díaita* means more than "diet." Indeed, the Greek word also communicates something along the lines of "way of life," or "mode of existence," or "lifestyle." The ancient Greek verb from which this word comes, διαιτάω, to "manage," or to "handle," further shows how closely connected this word is to "an approach to living." This matters because it reminds us that the Mediterranean lifestyle isn't just about food. The Mediterranean lifestyle is also about long walks on the beach, relaxing conversations with friends, ardent celebrations in the evening, and a general zest for full, present, passionate *being*. While the biological benefits derived from eating the constituent foods of the Mediterranean diet are well documented, I think it's worth remembering that any authentic path toward holistic health should include our bodies, minds, and souls. There's more to a "diet" than what we eat.

From a scientific perspective, the modern Mediterranean diet and its current practice really do place an enormous emphasis on *food*. The fame of the Mediterranean diet is the result of the work of Dr. Ancel Keys (1904–2004). Keys was a physiologist from Minnesota. He was also the first scientist to document the extraordinarily low incidence of cardiovascular disease in Mediterranean communities when compared to communities rooted in other areas of the world. Keys believed that diet was the primary determining factor in this comparison. Keys's famous study, published in 1970, was the result of research that he and his team carried out over ten years on over twelve thousand men from seven countries: Finland, Greece, Italy, Japan, Holland, the United States, and Yugoslavia. The results of this study are well known. Of these seven nations, Finland and the United States had the highest animal product consumption, the highest saturated fat intake, and the highest percentage of death from cardiovascular diseases. Japan, Italy, and Greece showed the exact opposite trends in terms of nutrition and mortality. The results of Keys's research have been confirmed consistently over the last fifty years. (The following chapters from Susan, Brynn, Shelby, and Mark give detailed summaries of recent research from their specific fields that confirm the well-known consensus that the Mediterranean diet is good for you.) With all that said, I've always thought that the *cultural* aspects of the Mediterranean diet are equally important and worthy of equal consideration and study. Indeed, while Keys is rightly renowned for his groundbreaking research on the link between diet and heart disease, there's no evidence that he ever emphasized the importance of the siesta, or *any* other cultural practice that defines Mediterranean life. This is entirely understandable, as this was not Keys's area of expertise or interest. But if we really want to understand the full scope of the Mediterranean diet, then we must ground this diet within its cultural and spiritual traditions.

This brings us to the midday nap. This brings us to the siesta.

The siesta—most famously associated with Greece, Italy, and Spain—has deep historical roots outside Western Europe. Indeed, the origins of the siesta can be traced to the most ancient civilizations of Asia, Africa, and the eastern Mediterranean. In the most basic terms, the midday nap seems to have been a simple, practical response to farm work in the afternoon heat. From there, it evolved into a set of longstanding cultural and religious traditions. Indeed, it's entirely possible that the siesta is as old as farming itself. If this is true, then the idea of the "formal, midday nap" probably has its origins in the Neolithic period. Even though there's no archaeological evidence for this practice during the Stone Age, common sense suggests that working outdoors, in the scalding midday sun would've been uncommon; our prehistoric ancestors felt and responded to blazing heat just like we do now. Interestingly, something like a siesta has been documented in the cases of numerous other primates. Red howler, rhesus, and white-faced capuchin monkeys, chimpanzees, and gorillas all nap after lunch and at other times. The primordial roots of this tradition seem firm.

During the historical period, more data is available. For example, in Pharaonic Egypt, it's entirely clear that workers and laborers followed a natural rhythm of work and rest dictated by the sun. We have very early evidence that farmers and slaves toiling in the Nile Delta paused during the peak heat, only to resume work in the cooler late afternoon. This practice was not confined to agricultural labor; it seems to have been a staple of all work, of any sort. There are several inscriptions from various temple building accounts dating between 2000 and 1500 BCE that suggest that a midday break was the norm. The famous Ebers Papyrus (c. 1550 BCE), an ancient Egyptian medical text, emphasizes the importance of midday rest for maintaining health in hot climates. Indeed, even Egyptian gods were believed to rest at noon. For example, the sun god Ra was thought to weaken during midday, symbolizing a time for humans to pause as well.

More evidence for the siesta comes from ancient Greece. Indeed, the ancient Greeks might have been the first among the Mediterranean civilizations to "formalize" the idea of a midday break for health reasons. This development seems to have been influenced by an interconnected matrix of common-sense climate awareness joined with a new-found interest in medicine and philosophy in the fifth and fourth centuries BCE. Of course, Greece's hot, dry summers made midday labor unbearable, particularly for farmers and outdoor workers. This reality is reflected by the ancient Greek writer Hesiod, who in his *Works and Days* (eighth century BCE) specifically advised that fieldwork should not be done during the peak heat of day; he recommended taking a nap instead. Much later, Hippocrates—the "Father of Western Medicine"—suggested that extreme heat disturbed the human body's balance. Hippocrates believed that maintaining a balance within the body, specifically a balance of the *four humors* (blood, phlegm, yellow bile, and black bile), was critical to health. A siesta would've been seen as a way to restore balance by allowing the body to rest and recover. Hippocrates also focused on scientifically observing the body and using natural and scientific medical remedies for healing rather than divine intervention. In this context, a siesta would've been considered a natural way to aid recovery and promote well-being. Indeed, in one of his most important writings, *On Regimen*, Hippocrates specifically recommends a mid-afternoon siesta as the way to both avoid imbalanced humors and to encourage well-being. Later, this idea was expanded by Aristotle who suggested that the real benefits of the siesta were mental rather than physical; the great thinker recommended an afternoon nap to restore clarity of mind.

The ancient Romans adopted and expanded the Greek custom of the siesta. Indeed, it's with the Romans that the siesta becomes a historically verifiable part of everyday commerce and everyday life. The Romans called their siesta the *meridiatio*. The word is derived from the Latin word *meridies*, or "midday." The break was taken around or just after noon, especially in rural areas, like clockwork. While Cato the Elder (234–149 BCE) wrote in *De Agricultura* that farmhands should rest during peak heat to prevent exhaustion, this practice was not confined to the countryside. The Roman poet Martial (first century BCE) pokes fun at wealthy city dwellers who take the enjoyment of a *post-prandium* (after-lunch) relaxation too far. In essence, by the time we get to the early empire, everyone in Rome was napping in the midafternoon, and by the time we get to the Renaissance, the modern version of the siesta—*riposo*—was firmly entrenched in Italian life.

In the post-Roman period, the traditional siesta is ubiquitous. During the Byzantine period, for example, the tradition was called the *hexapterygon* (six-hour pause), a practice that was adopted in Mediterranean monastic schedules that included rest after the "sixth hour," or noon. (The word *siesta* itself is derived from the Latin phrase "sexta hora.") In an identical fashion, the Islamic tradition of *qaylulah*—a short nap after the noon prayer, or *dhuhr*—spread the idea of the siesta from the eastern Mediterranean throughout the Islamic world. In fact, the siesta was specifically encouraged by the Prophet Muhammad who commanded: "Take short naps, for the devils do not take naps." Muhammad also noted: "Seek help in fasting by eating the pre-dawn meal and seek help in standing for night prayer by taking a nap during the day." This sacred wisdom was reiterated in classical Islamic medicine, as documented by Muslim scholars like the famous Avicenna (980–1037 CE) who recommended rest after the midday meal to aid digestion. During the Umayyad Caliphate (711–1492 CE), Islamic rulers in Spain introduced *qaylulah* to the Iberian Peninsula. This practice merged with local Visigothic and Roman customs, eventually evolving into what we now know as the classic, Mediterranean siesta.

Lest we trick ourselves into thinking that the siesta is only a "Mediterranean idea," or even a "European idea"—please do remember that the Chinese have a truly ancient tradition of post-lunch napping called *wǔjiào* and that the Japanese have an equally honored tradition of afternoon snoozing called *hirune*. In India and Nepal, the tradition is called *bhaat ghum*, which literally translates to "after-rice" sleep. In Vietnam, the tradition is called *ngủ trưa*, or "noon sleep." The siesta is an ancient, global, human tradition.

So, the siesta is an ancient idea.

But does that mean it's a *good* idea?

Here, modern research has added much.

One of the most noticeable and immediate benefits of taking an early afternoon nap is the enhancement of cognitive function. (It seems that Aristotle was right about this one!) Numerous studies have shown that a short nap of twenty to forty minutes can significantly boost alertness, concentration, and productivity, and that a little afternoon nap can make nappers more efficient and effective in their daily tasks. These benefits can be particularly helpful for those experiencing daytime sleepiness or grogginess due to poor sleep the night before. Moreover, taking early afternoon naps can significantly enhance our ability to learn and retain information. The benefits of napping include memory consolidation and improved problem-solving skills, making it easier to recall facts and details learned earlier in the day. This is particularly beneficial for students and professionals who need to absorb and retain a lot of information; it's also good for older folks. Most experts now agree that the brain uses the nap period to transfer information from short-term to long-term memory storage. Consequently, a brief nap can be an effective strategy for enhancing our capacity to learn and remember. In some cases, it can also enhance problem-solving abilities and stimulate creativity, making it a useful practice for those working in creative fields. How many times have you been told to "sleep on it?" There's real wisdom behind that guidance.

Another major advantage of the siesta that has been proven by modern science lies in the sphere of stress management. Chronic stress is a major contributor to various health problems, including cardiovascular disease and a weakened immune system. Afternoon naps are known to be effective in reducing stress and promoting relaxation. The post-lunch snooze triggers the release of serotonin (which helps to manage stress) and dopamine (which regulates mood and reduces feelings of anxiety). Additionally, the break from the day's demands and responsibilities during a nap allows the mind and body to relax, resulting in decreased levels of cortisol. Cortisol is the stress hormone; it's a killer. Anything that naturally reduces cortisol is going to be good for us.

Afternoon naps also have a mood-enhancing effect, which can be particularly valuable for people dealing with mood disorders or other emotional challenges/distress. The siesta can provide a much-needed emotional lift, particularly when you're feeling down or irritable. When we're well-rested, our emotional resilience is strengthened, making it easier to handle challenging situations. Taking our siestas can also reduce feelings of anger and hostility, fostering healthier relationships and better mental well-being. There's a reason we put little kids down for a nap in the afternoon. Nobody likes being crabby. The siesta can help fix this.

Of course, the benefits of early afternoon naps extend beyond cognitive and emotional well-being. Napping has been associated with improved cardiovascular health, too. Studies have shown that regular napping may help lower blood pressure and reduce the risk of heart disease, making it an important consideration for older adults and individuals at risk for cardiovascular issues. Napping promotes cardiovascular health by reducing stress and improving overall relaxation, which reduces the workload on the heart and decreases inflammation. Research from the American Heart Association has emphasized the potential cardiovascular benefits of incorporating daytime naps into our routines. More recently, it's been shown that a midday nap can reduce the risk of aneurysms. Researchers from the Lausanne University Hospital in Switzerland observed 3,400 people aged thirty-five to seventy-five for an average of five years. They discovered that those who napped once or twice per week had a lower risk of cardiovascular events in the brain. Moreover, a recent study from Dimitri Trichopoulos and his team noted that:

> There was a strong, duration-dependent and statistically significant association of afternoon sleep with the occurrence of (at least) non-fatal CHD episodes, indicating that a 30-minute siesta may be related with an almost 30 percent reduction of the corresponding incidence rate. Although the study is relatively small and residual confounding cannot be excluded, the results are not biologically implausible and appear remarkably consistent with the geocultural pattern of CHD occurrence (low incidence of CHD in siesta countries and population groups).

If this conclusion is true, then even this one, single benefit of the siesta would make it a worthwhile habit.

The siesta is also good for building a strong immune system. Early afternoon naps can serve as a valuable supplement to nighttime sleep, ensuring that our bodies get the rest they need for optimal function. When we're well-rested, our immune systems are better equipped to fight off illnesses and infections. Studies have shown that regular naps can help regulate the release of cytokines, which are proteins that play a key role in immune response. Siestas have also been shown to improve liver health. By bolstering your immune system, early afternoon naps can help you stay healthier and more resistant to diseases.

Several studies have suggested a link between regular napping and increased longevity. It appears that cultures where afternoon naps are commonplace have longer life expectancies. While napping alone is not a guarantee of a longer life, it may contribute to overall well-being and vitality, potentially leading to a healthier and longer life.

Finally, afternoon napping is *fun*—and it feels *good*. While my evidence is anecdotal, as a specialist in this particular area of research, my own experience with the siesta has been nothing but positive. And, if you have a partner who's also into the siesta, the potential benefits can compound quickly. Perhaps the time has come for all of us to get our naps on?

Chapter Two
Making Midwest Mediterranean Work for Busy Families—and Making Mealtimes Joyful for the Whole Family!

Megan Myrdal, MS, RD

I need to start my chapter with a confession–and an apology. As a registered dietitian who has provided guidance to individuals and families about healthy food choices for over fifteen years, I shared many thoughts and strategies during my single years that I thought were reasonable and doable for the typical working family. All of these ideas were backed by good scientific evidence on the food choices side but also were almost totally delusional regarding what it was actually like to feed small humans and oneself on a daily basis.

As a single woman for most of those years, I had all the time in the world and lots of notions about what was good, "practical" advice for parents and caregivers to make shopping, preparation, and mealtime optimal. Fast forward to my life today with a toddler, two elementary-aged stepsons, and my husband–that time is gone, and those notions have been shattered.

When I first started feeding my little family of five, I was filled with confidence about how I was going to do it–and how my kids would respond. I made lovely, balanced meals that were Midwest Mediterranean-focused while still being (what I perceived to be) kid-friendly. I served portions that I thought were appropriate for their age and size. And I offered at least one vegetable and fruit at each meal.

And what did I learn?

I learned that I was using tactics that I swore I never would, like "you have to eat *x* number of bites before you can leave the table." I learned that most meals ended with at least one child in tears over not wanting to eat the food. And I learned that I was tired, angry, and stressed because of the work I was putting in and the lack of enthusiasm (to put it lightly) for my cooking.

I needed to rethink my approach. I needed to let go of what I thought was "necessary" for my family's nutrition as well as my culinary skills and food knowledge. So, I got back to the basics of what research and parenting experts suggest are the best methods to feed families while incorporating Midwest Mediterranean ingredients as the foundation of our meals.

And what happened?

We approached the meals with less stress and concern over what we were eating and how it was going to be received. In all honesty, I was serving very similar food, just in a different format (less composed with more single ingredients—I'll say more on that later) and in a way that gave everyone more autonomy to pick what and how much he or she wanted. I was happier and present—able to focus more on the people I love and less on the foods we were eating, which is what mealtimes really should be about, right?

Before I share my experience and offer my advice on making family meals more joyful and less stressful based on the Midwest Mediterranean food principles, I'd like to start with a few notes and reflections:

First, most of what I'm sharing is based on my personal experiences as well as my reading and learning on the subject. I live in rural North Dakota and work to feed a family of five in a way that's healthy, balanced, low-stress, and budget-friendly. I personally feel that the Midwest Mediterranean dietary pattern works for our family, but I want to emphasize *pattern*. This is not our exclusive diet, and we definitely have foods in our house and on our table that are not prioritized in this way of eating; we also enjoy foods from other cultural traditions. We live in a global food system and are lucky to be able to enjoy foods and flavors from around the world. We keep a small garden in our backyard for produce that are staples in our household (tomatoes, onions, carrots, beets, squash) and shop at the weekly farmers market when it doesn't interfere with family activities. We do the bulk of our grocery shopping at supermarkets and big box stores and try to keep our pantry stocked with Midwest Mediterranean staples (extra-virgin olive oil, whole grains, canned beans, nuts, and seeds) for easy meal planning. We're omnivores and eat nearly all foods from all the food groups. We try to limit processed foods in our household, but we can't escape the occasional convenience of modern processed foods.

Second, families deal with a tremendous amount of food influence that originates outside our homes and develops our children's food preferences and habits. What children are offered at daycares and schools has a huge impact on what they like and want to eat. What they see their friends eating and what's provided when they visit other households also factors in. What they see on TV and social media has an impact. I know parents who try to hold their children accountable to only eating the "food code" they keep in their household, but I've rarely seen it work. Oftentimes it will create an increased desire for the "forbidden foods," with children putting excess attention on getting the off-limit foods. I hope that this chapter will provide some ideas for how you can offer and support healthy food choices without creating hard rules for your kids that will most likely backfire as they gain more freedom.

Third, the family eating style I am going to recommend is not without its skeptics. There are public health experts who say that this manner of feeding does not work in our modern food system, as the food environment is too unhealthy to have such a liberal approach to letting small humans feed themselves. I understand this. Childhood obesity is at an all-time high, with approximately one in five children and adolescents being clinically obese. For this dietary approach to reduce mealtime stress and create healthful eaters with healthy bodies, the food environment in the home also must be healthful, and children continually need to be offered a variety of healthful food choices that are emphasized in the Midwest Mediterranean diet. With that skepticism in mind, I will say that I believe this feeding method is the best way to develop a healthy, lifelong relationship with food. Our relationship with food shouldn't be obsessive or restrictive. We should teach our children to care for their bodies and to eat in a way that nourishes them, but we should also teach them about the pleasure and enjoyment in eating—to which we know good, delicious food can contribute so much!

Finally, what I'm going to share may not be an overnight revolution in your family's dietary habits. If your household foods have predominantly been hot dogs and macaroni and cheese, simply presenting Midwest Mediterranean foods in my suggested manner isn't going to magically make them desirable to your family. It takes time. It takes baby steps. It takes repeated exposure—research says about 15–20+ times! It takes patience. Good luck!

Okay, now into the "meat" of my chapter.

How do you make Midwest Mediterranean work for your busy family while maintaining your sanity?

First, I'd like to start with *how* to feed your family, then we'll move to *what* to feed them.

The *how* is a revolutionary concept that was developed in the 1980s called "The Divisions of Responsibility."

The Divisions of Responsibility

One of the foremost experts on childhood feeding is a registered dietitian named Ellyn Satter. She runs the Ellyn Satter Institute and famously developed the Divisions of Responsibility when it comes to childhood feeding.

What are the "Divisions of Responsibility?" Simply put, the Divisions of Responsibility lay out who in the household (parent or child) is responsible for what aspects of feeding and eating.

According to Ellyn, parents are responsible for the *what*, *where*, and *when*, and kids are responsible for the *if* and *how much*.

What does this mean? It means that, as the parent, I determine *what* we're eating (chicken, beans, pasta, and roasted broccoli), *where* we're eating it (the kitchen table), and *when* we're eating (6 p.m.), and the kids are responsible for *if* they eat and *how much* they eat of the different foods. So, the child can decide to eat all or none of the food, and they choose to eat however much of each food they like. This part gets concerning for many parents because they worry that if their child only eats the noodles and not the rest of the food items, their nutrition will suffer. The institute's research confirms that continued offering and not pressuring is the route to get kids to like and eat different foods and to develop lifelong healthy food patterns, and that the small nutritional gaps during this time are inconsequential. Pressure or coercion doesn't work. Continuing to offer, encourage, and support healthful eating does.

We switched to this style of eating about a year ago, and the boys loved it immediately. You could instantly see the joy on their faces because they were in control of these aspects of their eating experience. Also, giving children age-appropriate choices helps them develop their decision-making skills, feel a sense of control, and learn independence. Mealtimes are a wonderful opportunity for young people to grow and flex these skills while exposing them to the incredible array of healthy, delicious foods, such as those in the Midwest Mediterranean diet.

I know what many of you might be thinking as you read this: SO MANY DISHES! Yes, there are a few more dishes to clean doing family meals in this way. I try to use serving containers that have a lid, so I can simply put the leftovers in the fridge when we're finished. I've also found that the kids get a kick out of "charcuterie-style" dinners, so if we're having (for example) a grilled meat, roasted carrots, and toasted bread for dinner, I might put it all on a large cutting board and set it in the middle of the table for serving. I try to remind myself that a few more dishes are much easier to manage than a dinner table meltdown. This style of eating is typically done during the evening meal in our household, or "supper" as we call it in the Midwest. It can absolutely be done for breakfast and lunch, but we typically eat very similar foods for those meals (oatmeal, yogurt, eggs, fresh fruit, sandwiches, wraps, etc.) and are usually a little more rushed at those meals, so dinner is our occasion to use this eating style and introduce new foods.

Also, I must note that we don't do this for every evening meal. My husband and I both work full-time, and the kids are busy with many activities that come close to the evening eating hour. There are days when it's a time challenge to simply get dinner on the table—let alone have it plated in this manner. Have grace with yourself and be happy doing the best you can!

(You also might be wondering: *How do I do snacks with this style of eating?* The Divisions of Responsibility allows for snacks, but it encourages that snacks should not be so appetizing that kids forgo their meal to wait for their beloved snack. Midwest Mediterranean snacks that we enjoy frequently in our household are whole grain crackers with cheese, fresh fruit, vegetables with dip, nuts, trail mix, hard-boiled eggs, lower sugar yogurt, and whole grain bread with nut butter. The kids know these are the snack options in our household, and they like them, but not so much that they crave them.)

To read more about this eating pattern, I recommend checking out one of the numerous books Ms. Satter has written, as well as the Ellyn Satter Institute website to learn more.

Now that we've talked about *how* to present the foods, let's talk about *what* your family should eat if you want to follow the Midwest Mediterranean diet.

I should note that the work of the Ellyn Satter Institute doesn't recommend specific foods or portions and encourages eaters to develop their own competence for food that agrees with their lifestyle and bodies. I tend to agree with this philosophy, and my following recommendations aren't meant to be prescriptive or absolute. I find many parents are hungry for meal ideas and recipe recommendations, so I hope the following guidelines are helpful; all can be modified based on your family's needs.

The Mediterranean diet is based on the traditional dietary pattern of people who live in the countries that surround the Mediterranean Sea. Decades of research on the diet consistently shows that people who eat in this way age more healthfully and have a lower risk of cardiovascular disease as well as an increased lifespan. The diet emphasizes:

- **an abundance of plant foods including whole grains, legumes (beans, peas, lentils, and chickpeas), fruits, vegetables, and nuts—ideally those that are minimally processed and locally grown**
- **olive oil as the principal fat**
- **cheese and yogurt, consumed daily in low to moderate amounts**
- **fish and poultry, consumed in low to moderate amounts a few times a week**
- **wine consumed in low to moderate amounts, usually with meals (obviously for those 21+)**
- **infrequent consumption of red meat, refined grains, and sweets**

As we discuss here and in our previous book, the Midwest Mediterranean diet encourages eating like a Mediterranean but also consuming Midwest staples like potatoes, wild rice, sunflower seeds, freshwater fish, and utilizing preservation techniques like canning, pickling, and fermentation to extend the life of our local, seasonal foods into the winter months.

As we look at this food list, there are ample foods that kids love, but also some that are a little more foreign.

What I've learned in my trials and errors in feeding my family a Midwest Mediterranean-style diet is that it's important to have familiar favorites at each meal while continuing to offer new options. Familiar favorites are the foods that your kids will always eat. It might be noodles with olive oil, rice with mixed vegetables, roasted potatoes, whole grain bread, grilled chicken tenders, etc. What I've found works best in our household is to serve several simple food options that people can enjoy individually or build together into a more complex dish. Parents don't want to suffer through the monotony of eating plain noodles at every meal, and most kids aren't yet interested in the complex flavors and textures that are traditional of the Midwest Mediterranean diet. This strategy offers a simple and pragmatic solution.

Here are a few examples of what I mean.

Dinner Idea #1:

- **cooked pasta with extra-virgin olive oil**
- **shrimp sauteed in extra-virgin olive oil**
- **roasted broccoli**
- **cherry tomatoes**
- **pistachios**

This is a meal you will frequently see on our dinner table. All the options are served individually at the dinner table, each person gets to pick what they want, and each person gets to pick how much of each option they want. My husband and I will eat everything, likely mixing it together for a bowl-type dish, possibly adding a little more olive oil, balsamic vinegar, and some feta cheese. The kids will each pick what they want. They will always take the pasta and cherry tomatoes—and sometimes the shrimp, broccoli, and pistachios. As time has gone by and we continue to do this, they've become more receptive to the other foods. Research has shown that the single most effective strategy in getting kids to eat new foods is *repeated exposure*. They may need to try something 15–20 times before they know if they like it or not. As foods are continually offered, they become more familiar. And with familiarity comes acceptance.

Here is another example of a Midwest Mediterranean family meal.

Dinner Idea #2:

- **chicken meatballs**
- **whole grain pitas**
- **shredded spinach**
- **cherry tomatoes**
- **sliced cucumbers**
- **sliced red onion**
- **tzatziki sauce**

Again, my husband and I will eat everything, likely making a falafel-style meatball sandwich, whereas the kids might just eat meatballs, cherry tomatoes, and sliced cucumbers. Again, it's all on the table and available. They see us eating it. They are exposed to it. But there's no pressure or coercion. Simple exposure and offering.

Dinner Idea #3:

- **whole grain couscous with olive oil and salt**
- **sliced chicken breast**
- **roasted chickpeas**
- **avocado**
- **shredded spinach**
- **corn**
- **peanuts**
- **Midwest Mediterranean ranch (see recipe in Appendix A)**

Kids' choice: likely couscous, chicken, corn, peanuts, and ranch.

Parents' choice: bowls with everything, likely adding a little hot sauce for a kick!

Are you seeing the picture and the pattern?

A few notes for these foods:

> ***Pasta***: This is our top familiar favorite. Our kids love pasta, and luckily there is such a range of pasta products available today. There are many delicious pasta options that utilize more nutrient-dense ingredients like lentils, peas, or beans; are whole grain; and/or are made with crop varieties that are higher in protein and fiber than traditional durum wheat. I encourage you to spend a little extra time in the pasta aisle on your next shopping trip and see if you find a new product that appeals to your family. Also, pasta is a wonderful way to get your kids to love extra-virgin olive oil!
>
> ***Roasting vegetables***: Our family *loves* roasted vegetables. I love to batch cook large quantities of roasted broccoli, carrots, potatoes, brussels sprouts, and cauliflower, and keep them in the fridge for quick meal additions. Roasting brings out amazing flavor in vegetables, and using extra-virgin olive oil

adds an extra layer of nutrition to these powerhouse vegetables for your family.

Proteins: Try to vary your proteins between animal and non-animal. Beans, peas, and lentils are your friends—and are grown in abundance in the Midwest! Canned tuna and salmon can be lifesavers for quick meals. Also, rotisserie chicken is a great option in a pinch!

Canned Beans: We're a big canned bean household and keep all types of canned beans in our pantry for quick, easy meal additions. If you're currently cooking dried beans, kudos and keep it up! If you are looking for simple ways to get your kids to eat more beans, try roasting chickpeas to bring out great flavor and a crunchy texture (add a little extra-virgin olive oil and salt and roast at 425°F for 20–30 minutes) or pureeing black beans with a little olive oil, lemon juice, cumin, garlic, salt, and pepper into a delicious hummus for fresh vegetables!

Healthy Fats: Use extra-virgin olive oil from a trusted source as your main fat and enjoy avocados, nuts, and seeds regularly.

Fruit: We try to keep a nice assortment of fresh, seasonal fruit in our house and serve it with all meals. I find it tempting to continue buying the same fruits over and over, because I know the kids will eat them, but I try to challenge myself to buy just one different item each week. It might be one plum, mango, or pear—simply as an opportunity for the kids to try it. If they like it and want more, I'll buy more.

A few fast, final notes on making Midwest Mediterranean work for busy families:

Meal Prepping! Meal prepping goes a long way in making mealtimes less stressful and more enjoyable for all. If you can spend a couple hours on a weekend prepping ingredients like chopped vegetables, cooked grains (e.g., quinoa, farro), and grilled proteins (chicken, fish), it goes a long way in making the weeknight meals more enjoyable.

Everyone Loves to Dip! Kids love to dip almost everything they eat into a tasty condiment, and I must confess, I do too! However, finding condiments that aren't made with 30+ ingredients and numerous additives and preservatives is challenging. In the recipe section of this book, you'll find my recipe for Midwest Mediterranean Ranch—because what Midwesterner can live without ranch dressing?! It's made with Greek yogurt and an array of spices and can easily last for two weeks in the fridge. It's tasty, nutritious, and makes many vegetables more appetizing for palates both young and old!

Picky Eating? Picky eating is totally normal as kids go through different stages of development. One day they might love oranges and the next day they hate them. Try not to get overly stressed or upset. Continue with the plan—one day at a time, and offering, never pressuring.

Stock the Pantry! Keep a well-stocked Midwest Mediterranean pantry with items like extra-virgin olive oil (always from a trusted source), canned beans, whole grains (quinoa, brown or wild rice, whole grain pasta), canned tomatoes, nuts, seeds, herbs, and spices.

Get Everyone Involved! Encourage everyone to get involved by having family cooking night! Assign age-appropriate tasks like mixing dry ingredients (three years and older), setting the table (four years and older), washing fruits and vegetables and measuring ingredients (six to eight years old), and reading the recipe and demonstrating safe knife skills (nine and older).

I hope this chapter has provided some new ideas, and/or reinforced the good work you're already doing in your household kitchen. Again, I don't promise instant results, but I believe over time that feeding your family in this way, and with these foods, is a wonderful foundation to develop a healthy, joyful relationship with food—and the Midwest Mediterranean!

Chapter Three
Midwest Wine Reimagined

Sean N. Ballinger

Midwest wine has long grappled with a reputation built on provincial myths and thus is often dismissed as overly sweet, acidic, and reliant on fruit like rhubarb and chokecherries. While there is historical truth to this mythology, the industry is currently engaged in a renaissance. The production of Midwest wine is now more in line with those of other traditional wine regions. I have witnessed this transformation and the unique potential of cold-climate grapes firsthand. My first encounter with fine wine from the Midwest was in 2012 when I tasted a dry red made from the Petite Pearl grape. That wine, beautifully balanced and traditional in style, surprised me not just with its quality but with its origin—the grapes had been grown on my family's estate on the outskirts of Fargo, North Dakota! That tasting reshaped the trajectory of my life. I found myself captivated by the potential of cold-climate grapes and chose to devote my professional life to winemaking. It's well known that high quality wine consumed in moderation forms one pillar of the Mediterranean diet. In this chapter, I'm going to examine the history, nature, and potential of Midwest wine and its relationship to the Mediterranean tradition.

The Evolution of a Wine Region

Wine regions transition from infancy, defined by innovation and discovery, to maturity, characterized by tradition and preservation. In the early stages, winemakers focus on discovering the unique flavors and qualities their terroir can produce, while mature regions work to protect and maintain those established identities. Today, the Midwest is in its exploratory phase, with winemakers striving to define what this region can and should taste like. My hope is that future generations, including my grandchildren, will inherit a wine region where the terroir we are uncovering today becomes a legacy they cherish and preserve.

Preservation vs. Discovery: Contrasting Wine Philosophies

Modern Mediterranean winemakers are the stewards of centuries-old traditions. They preserve what their ancestors perfected, adhering to established rules dictating everything from grape varieties and harvest timing to fermentation methods and aging periods. This approach safeguards their reputation and ensures consistency for international audiences—but it often limits innovation. In contrast, the philosophy of Midwest winemaking is one of relentless experimentation. Here, tradition is nearly non-existent, and clinging to the past means being left behind. The US wine laws are far less restrictive than those of the Mediterranean, granting Midwest winemakers the freedom to plant, ferment, and create without constraint. While California wineries enjoy similar freedoms, as a region, they have entered the preservation stage, focusing on maintaining their reputation rather than pushing boundaries. Both the preservation and discovery mindsets have value in the world of wine. Preservation honors history and identity, while discovery drives innovation and creativity. Together, they create a dynamic and diverse global wine landscape.

Redefining Tradition through Cold-Climate Grapes

The transformation of Midwest wine into a fine wine contender is rooted in a long-standing tradition of grape breeding. While grapes from the Mediterranean, such as Merlot and Chardonnay, belong to the renowned *Vitis vinifera* species and thrive in temperate climates, these varieties would freeze in the harsh winters of the Midwest. Fortunately, *Vitis vinifera* is not the only grapevine species. In fact, there are between sixty and one hundred grapevine species worldwide (depending on the source), many of which are native to the frigid climates of the Americas. Two of the most significant American species are *Vitis riparia* and *Vitis labrusca*, which naturally thrive in cold climates. The goal of cold-climate grape breeding has been to blend the resilience of these American species with the refined flavor profiles of *Vitis vinifera*. The result? Hardy grape varieties capable of withstanding extreme Midwest conditions while producing wines reminiscent of their Mediterranean counterparts.

The esteemed status of *Vitis vinifera* is evident in its nicknames: the “noble grape” and the “wine grape.” It dominates winemaking, accounting for 99 percent of all wine produced globally. A quick glance at any wine shop reveals its ubiquity, with varieties like merlot, Sangiovese, sauvignon blanc, and chardonnay filling the shelves. For most casual wine drinkers, naming a grape that is not pure *Vitis vinifera* would be a challenge. Yet, this *vinifera*-centric perspective, often championed by wine purists, is both limited and outdated. A bias toward the familiar and lack of access to non-*vinifera* wines have likely fueled this perception. As Midwest wines continue to innovate and gain recognition, they will challenge these traditional notions, proving that excellence in winemaking can emerge from unexpected places, even amid the snow and soil of the Midwest.

A Tale of Two Continents: The Evolution of Grapevines

Around eighty-five million years ago, during the era of the supercontinent Pangea, a single type of grapevine thrived across the northern hemisphere. As Pangea fractured and landmasses drifted apart, this primitive vine diversified into multiple species, each adapting to unique environments. *Vitis vinifera*, the species responsible for nearly all fine wines, evolved in Europe and Asia, while species like *Vitis labrusca* and *Vitis riparia* developed in North America. Over millions of years, these species acquired distinct characteristics: *Vitis labrusca* is known for its "foxy," grapey flavor, reminiscent of Welch's grape juice, while *Vitis riparia* developed high acidity and remarkable cold hardiness, enabling it to endure extreme climates. These evolutionary differences not only shaped their flavors but also their ability to thrive in vastly different environments, laying the foundation for modern grape breeding.

Elmer Swenson: The Godfather of Midwest Wine

Within this context of hardy grape varieties, the legacy of Wisconsin grape breeder Elmer Swenson (1913–2004) must be mentioned. Often called "the godfather of Midwest wine," Swenson's impact on our region's viticulture is immeasurable. Ironically, Swenson rarely drank wine himself—his initial goal was to breed cold-hardy grapes for eating, not winemaking. It was those around him who recognized the Dionysian potential in his work. Over a prolific fifty-year career, Swenson released eighteen named grape varieties, four of which I use today: St. Pepin, Brianna, Prairie Star, and Louise Swenson. While this timeline may seem modest compared to regions where grape varieties boast centuries or even millennia of history, in the Midwest—where the hunt for the "new grape" dominates—Swenson's creations have stood the test of time quite well, solidifying his status as a pioneer in cold-climate viticulture.

Elmer Swenson's most groundbreaking achievement was drastically reducing the acidity of cold-climate grapes, making it possible to produce dry table wines that are balanced and not overwhelmingly tart. Building on Elmer's legacy, his student—and my mentor—Tom Plocher refined this innovation, focusing on dry red wines and selecting exceptional varieties like Crimson Pearl, Petite Pearl, Verona, and Veritage, with more on the horizon. At Bear Creek Winery, Crimson Pearl has become a flagship grape, earning local respect and showcasing the potential of cold-hardy grapes. Tom's career has centered on perfecting a single style of wine, dry reds. I find his discipline inspiring! He has been generous enough to send dozens of his experimental varieties to Bear Creek for evaluation, and several have shown great promise.

A Tribute to the Universities

While Tom Plocher has made remarkable advances in cold-climate grape breeding, universities have also been instrumental in shaping Midwest viticulture. The University of Minnesota, a leader in the field since Elmer Swenson's era, has developed groundbreaking varieties like Frontenac (noir and gris), Marquette, La Crescent, Itasca, and Clarion, each introducing distinct flavors and styles to the region. However, for areas with harsher winters and shorter growing seasons, like North Dakota, further innovation has been needed. In response, my father, Rod Ballinger, and others founded the North Dakota State University Grape Germplasm Enhancement Project, which is now poised to release its own hardy white varieties, Radiant and Dakota Primus, paving the way for the next chapter in Midwest winemaking.

Naming Midwest Grapes

Over the years, various names have been proposed for our northern grape varieties: "cold-resistant grapes," "cold-hardy grapes," "hybrids," "inter-specific hybrids," "northern grapes," and my personal favorite, "cold-climate grapes." While a bit wordy, this term best captures the essence of these grapes across all four seasons. Other names focus too heavily on scientific terminology or emphasize winter conditions, overlooking the full story. In Europe, discussions about cold-climate wine often revolve around summer challenges, like shorter growing seasons, since winters are irrelevant for dormant vines. However, in the Midwest, winter dieback is a critical factor, making the term "cold-climate grapes" fitting for both the growing season and the harsh winters that shape these vines's resilience and character.

Tannin and Cold-Climate Grapes

The Midwest produces a diverse array of wine styles, many achievable with cold-climate grapes. However, one style remains elusive: the high-tannin, full-bodied dry red wines that Mediterranean vineyards have perfected. Notable examples include Brunello (Tuscany), Priorat (Spain), Châteauneuf-du-Pape (Southern Rhône), Nero d'Avola (Sicily), Xinomavro (Greece), and my personal favorite, Barolo (Piedmont).

While many Midwest wineries feature locally grown dry reds on their menus, these wines are typically smoother and lighter in body, comparable to pinot noir. This is largely due to the low tannin levels found in cold-climate grape varieties. Tannins—polyphenols located in the seeds, skins, and stems of grapes—contribute astringency, structure, and age-ability, often considered the backbone of robust red wines. For Midwest winemakers, their absence is omnipresent. For generations, grape breeders have been on the hunt for the elusive "tannin bomb" cold-climate grape. After tackling acidity, increasing tannin levels has become the next big goal. While progress has been made, the ultimate breakthrough remains just out of reach, leaving winemakers eager to see what the future holds for Midwest reds.

Cold Climate Limited to White Wine?

Tannin levels in white wines are far less significant than in reds, as the seeds and skins are removed before fermentation. Instead, acidity is the backbone of white wine, giving it structure and vibrancy. Considering the Midwest's low tannin levels, relatively high acidity, and short growing season, it would be tempting to assume that white wines are destined to dominate the region. Historically, this has been the case for cold climates—think of the German monks in the Middle Ages who crafted renowned Rieslings but struggled to earn acclaim for their reds. This historical precedent has guided vintners globally, especially those working with *Vitis vinifera*.

But does it apply to cold-climate grapes?

The answer requires a closer look at key variables, particularly the length of the growing season. White wine grapes typically thrive in cooler climates, where their earlier ripening suits shorter seasons. This has often made white wines the logical choice for regions with challenging growing conditions. However, cold-climate grapes, bred specifically for harsh environments, ripen faster than vinifera. Despite this, in difficult vintages, we still often struggle to fully ripen our red varieties. That said, the future looks promising. This year, I witnessed something remarkable: An experimental red grape developed by Tom Plocher, known as TP-4-4-40, reached full maturity a month before the fall frost—even in a cold vintage. Incredibly, we harvested it earlier than many white varieties. This milestone suggests that the next generation of cold-climate red grapes will ripen reliably, even in challenging conditions, opening the door for reds to consistently flourish alongside whites in the upper Midwest.

In Defense of Midwest Sweet Wine

I have a saying: "Wine drinkers go through three stages of development. First, they solely drink sweet wine. Then, they solely drink dry wine. Finally, they drink both." The final stage is marked by the ability to see beauty in all styles of wine and a curiosity to experience every possible flavor.

Sweet wine has a long-standing history in the Midwest, and this is no accident. The style aligns wonderfully with the region's grapes, climate, and culture. High acidity is effectively balanced by sugar. Despite the energy devoted to the new grape varieties that lend themselves to dry wine, a significant number of grapes still planted in the area require sugar to achieve balance. As long as the sugar levels remain within respectable levels, these wines can still taste delicious and sell exceptionally well.

Sweet wines also pair beautifully with certain dishes, particularly those with spice. The lack of sweetness in wine can make them taste overly astringent when paired with umami-rich foods. This factor suggests sweet wines will have significance going forward.

Sweet wines often carry a stigma, with the notable exception of fortified wines. Typically, fortified wines are very sweet; despite this, the wine is perceived as a sophisticated beverage by wine enthusiasts. I believe this is due to the brandy and barrel reducing the fruity character of the wine. Moreover, the wine's high alcohol levels allow it to age gracefully for decades. So if low tannin levels prove inhibitory to a wine's aging potential, this style could be the Midwest's ticket to age-worthy wines.

The Age-Ability of Cold-Climate Wines

One of the hallmarks of fine wine is its ability to age gracefully. But what determines a wine's aging potential? It comes down to a wine's chemical composition and the conditions in which it is stored. Traditional wine regions, where grapes and wines have been tested across countless vintages, benefit from centuries of experience, creating a reliable understanding of how wines evolve over time. In contrast, the Midwest's winemaking tradition is still in its infancy. Our grape varieties and wineries are relatively new, meaning we haven't had generations to observe how these wines mature. However, there are chemical indicators that suggest cold-climate wines may age as successfully as *vinifera*-based wines. The key traits of age-worthy wines—high acidity, tannin, and complexity in youth—are all present in many cold-climate grapes.

At Bear Creek Winery, we've created an experimental wine cellar to study the aging potential of cold-climate wines. By cellaring wines we believe have aging potential, we're building a body of evidence to understand their evolution over decades. Some of these wines, now up to twenty years old, are showing beautifully, with flavors deepening and maturing in remarkable ways. Others haven't stood the test of time and have been relegated to the drain. This ongoing experiment allows us to uncover which varieties and styles age best, offering exciting possibilities for the future of Midwest winemaking.

The Future of Midwest Wine

What wines will be grown in the Midwest in one hundred years? What flavors will winemakers be able to achieve? What styles will define our region? Will bold reds rival those of Napa, or will entirely new expressions emerge, rooted in our unique terroir? As a winemaker, I cannot help but wonder if my predictions will come close—or if future generations will craft something so extraordinary that it surpasses anything we can imagine today. My perspective on this issue shifts constantly—chilly summers convince me white wine is the future, but a barrel tasting of a great red makes me rethink everything. At farmers markets, where sweet wines dominate, my predictions shift again. This constant cycle of doubt and discovery highlights the complexity of Midwest winemaking. To move forward, we must learn from the Mediterranean's success—what makes their wines so timelessly seductive? By crafting flavors that balance familiarity with innovation, we can let the community shape the region's identity. However, if we grow complacent or cling to the past, Midwest wine will fail to achieve its full potential. My hope is that the terroir we strive to discover today becomes a legacy for future generations to preserve and celebrate.

Chapter Four
The Greek Approach to the Sweet Life

Susan Mathison, MD

In ancient times, the Greeks relied on honey as a sweetener in their diet. Honey was a common ingredient in various dishes and also prized for its medicinal properties. Greeks enjoyed fruits, both fresh and dried, like figs, dates, and raisins, which provided natural sweetness. Modern Greeks embrace desserts as an integral part of their culinary and cultural traditions, balancing sweetness with a focus on natural and high-quality ingredients. Desserts are associated with hospitality. Offering sweets to guests is a long-standing tradition, symbolizing warmth and generosity.

Afternoon or evening guests are sometimes offered spoon sweets, which are fruits preserved in a sugary syrup. In ancient times, wine and honey were used to make the syrup. Sour cherries, oranges, figs, tomatoes, nuts, and even rose petals have been used to make delicate spoon sweets. These are served from the jar onto tiny plates, often with a matching spoon, and accompanied by coffee and a glass of cold water.

Baked desserts like *baklava*, *kataifi*, and *ravani* are still popular, especially during holidays and celebrations. *Melomakarona* (honey-drenched cookies) and *kourabiedes* (buttery almond cookies) are staples during Christmas. *Tsoureki* is a sweet bread for Easter, and *vasilopita* is a cake served on New Year's Day with a hidden coin for luck.

Greek yogurt with honey and walnuts or fresh fruit serve as simple, healthy dessert options.

Modern Greeks, much like people in many other countries, are becoming increasingly health-conscious and aware of the impact of processed sugar on health. Greece has the highest obesity rate in Europe, though still a lower rate than in the US. With the global availability of processed and packaged foods, consumption of sugary snacks and drinks has increased, particularly among Greek children and teens.

Public health campaigns in Greece emphasize reducing sugar intake and adopting healthier eating habits.

The biochemical damage caused by sugar primarily involves its impact on metabolic processes and cellular functions. Excessive sugar intake can lead to increased levels of glucose in the bloodstream, resulting in a large production of insulin from the beta cells of the pancreas. Other cells become less responsive to insulin, and the beta cells have a hard time keeping up with demands for more insulin and eventually fail. This can initiate a cascade of metabolic disorders, including type 2 diabetes, cardiovascular disease, cerebrovascular disease, and even cancer.

High sugar consumption is linked to the production of advanced glycation end products (AGEs), which can damage proteins, lipids, and DNA, contributing to inflammation and oxidative stress. This process can accelerate aging and increase the risk of chronic diseases mentioned above. Think of it as caramelized rust deposits on important structures that eventually destroy their function. An example would be an elderly person with a textured, leather-like appearance of the skin from deep, crisscrossed wrinkles. Foot neuropathy and visual impairment are other examples of glycation.

Even when we understand the potential harm of overindulging, the excess sugar habit can be hard to break. Sweet foods activate dopamine release in the brain, stimulating feelings of pleasure and satisfaction. These good feelings make us want more, to the point of cravings and even addiction. It's said that sugar is more addictive than cocaine, yet it legally surrounds us. Marketing agencies for food products cleverly dial up our cravings with their ad campaigns. Getting excess sugar out of our diets is even more of a challenge when we have withdrawal symptoms like headaches and shakiness for several days when we stop eating it.

Thankfully, the Mediterranean diet, which emphasizes fresh, whole foods, naturally discourages excessive consumption of refined sugar and starches. Depending on the region, Greek meals usually incorporate fresh vegetables, fresh fish or meat, and a generous dose of olive oil. If dessert is served, it tends to be eaten in moderation at the end of a meal. From a nutritional point of view, the Mediterranean diet goes *very* easy on the sugar. It's hard to overstate the importance of this fact. Indeed, if you want to do one thing—and one thing only—to make yourself feel better, do what the Mediterraneans do and reduce your intake of sugar.

Timing is helpful for minimizing the metabolic impact of dessert, even if it is made with refined sugar. By eating vegetables, protein, and healthy fats, such as olive oil, before refined carbohydrates, the blood glucose spike we experience is modulated to a level 30 to 40 percent lower than what it would be if the carbs were eaten on their own or first. This steadying effect can be prolonged even further by walking at a leisurely pace for just ten minutes or doing some extra movement as you clean up because the muscles take up glucose for fuel as they move. You can read more about these simple hacks from Dr. Jessie Inchauspe, author of *Glucose Revolution* and *The Glucose Goddess Method*.

Many Greeks, especially younger generations, are more mindful of limiting sugar intake and reading labels to avoid hidden sugars in processed foods. The Nova system is a globally recognized classification that will make deciphering labels easier, since we can scan the product's bar code for information. Nova was developed with the idea that knowing the extent and purpose of processing applied to different foods can help explain the relationship between health, disease, and dietary patterns. The system has been used as a common framework for grouping foods and beverages depending on the level of processing, with Group 1 being a whole food, such as an apple, and Group 4 being an ultra-processed food, like a fast-food fried apple pie. In US grocery stores, 72 percent of the products sold are considered to be ultra-processed and unhealthy.

A new update of the Nova classification system will aim to make it more helpful by taking the nutritional content of foods into account for scoring; it should be ready by 2026.

Increased awareness and a focus on moderation allow sweets and desserts to remain an integral part of Greek culture, often enjoyed during celebrations or with coffee after a meal.

Many Greeks appreciate the effort to minimize processed sugar in recipes, and there's a growing market for sugar-free or low-sugar products. Artificial sweeteners are available but can have harmful biologic effects. There are some natural, but minimally caloric, sweeteners like stevia, monkfruit, and allulose that may be safely incorporated into traditional Greek desserts without removing their tasty allure. I've included a Greek almond cookie recipe in Appendix A that uses almond flour, monkfruit, and allulose and produces a delicious and authentic result without inducing a large spike in blood sugar.

Greeks also have the advantage of a slower pace at mealtimes. Instead of life in the fast lane with fast food, Greeks seem to savor their meals. Smaller bites, more chewing, and more socializing adds up to a healthier lifestyle. By slowing down, digestion improves, and food seems more satisfying. Weight management becomes easier since you notice when you are full more easily.

Maybe you don't need dessert? But if you do, be mindful of the options described above—and then truly enjoy it!

Chapter Five
The Mediterranean See: Eyes, Diet, and Vision

Brynn Peterson, BA, OD

Before there were eyes to see, there was light. From the first time cellular life wiggled out of the steaming muck and survived the noxious environment it called home, it was able to capture sunlight so it could be transferred to energy for the cell. This conversion of light was made possible because retinal—a form of vitamin A—combined with a protein—opsin—to form *rhodopsin*. Thus, the rhodopsin family of proteins has been in existence for literally millennia, allowing for light utilization or "sight."

From an anthropocentric position, rhodopsin is commonly identified as being an integral protein in the retina, helping with vision in dim or dark conditions. This is a relatively recent development, however, as humans are newcomers to earth's historical timeline. Though its origins are ancient, today vitamin A is known to be an integral component for ocular and systemic health; not having enough can lead to many problems. Today we get vitamin A from many dietary sources such as milk, cheese, eggs, yogurt, fish, leafy greens, and tomatoes.

This abbreviated historical account of rhodopsin and vitamin A is meant to emphasize the idea that while some things become obsolescent, some things never do—like the Mediterranean diet. In a society always looking for the latest wellness trend or medical "fix," sometimes it is prudent to remember the wisdom of history. The same building blocks that helped the first life on earth utilize light to "see" are some of the same we rely upon today for good ocular health. Thus, it is important that we tailor our diet for optimal health and wellness. Although it may not herald back to prehistoric times, the evidence supporting this diet's enhancement of overall well-being is more abundant every year.

Vision is complex. It involves (ideally) both eyes working together. It requires many different parts of the eye each working properly to have clear and comfortable vision. It involves the optic nerve from each eye winding through multiple areas of the brain and meeting in the occipital lobe, located in the back of the brain near where the spine meets the skull. It is here in the occipital lobe of the brain that visual perception and processing take place. Thus, when we think of sight, we are not only thinking of ocular health but also neurologic health.

Because vision is so complex and there are so many different components of excellent vision, there are many variables that can affect ocular function and many things that can go wrong at any point in the visual pathway. Just as it is with any other aspect of our lives, it is most productive to focus on the things we can do and the things we have control over. Or, as we say in healthcare, "modifiable risk factors." One of the most accessible things we can do—besides throwing on sunglasses when we are outdoors and avoiding tobacco products—is intentionally eat good food. This means diet. And this brings us to Midwest Mediterranean.

Meibomian Gland Dysfunction:
Why are my eyes watering if they are dry?

In our first stop through the visual system, at the front surface of the eye, we will consider the eyelids and tear film. A robust, evenly distributed tear film across the front of the eye is imperative for clear and comfortable vision. Without a healthy tear film, patients can experience a myriad of unpleasant symptoms such as irritation, burning, foreign body sensation, redness, and blurred vision. There are different types of dry eye and many different causes of dryness, from autoimmune disease to hormonal changes and aging, long-term contact lens wear and refractive surgery, localized inflammation of the eyelids, and vitamin deficiencies.

One of the most prevalent types of dryness is evaporative dry eye from meibomian gland dysfunction (MGD). The meibomian glands line the upper and lower eyelids and produce the oily layer of our tear film, meibum. This oily layer prevents the watery layer of our tear film, produced by the lacrimal gland, from evaporating and helps to keep our tears evenly distributed across the eye. Without it, people notice that their eyes reflexively water as their tears are evaporating too quickly, especially outdoors in the wind. It is a seemingly paradoxical side effect, to which people inquire, "How can my eyes be dry if they are watering uncontrollably?" Often, these watery tears are a momentary solution of the body, but do not provide a stable tear film that provides real relief. People may also note that their vision fluctuates greatly, especially when looking at electronic devices as blink rate decreases markedly when looking at screens. And sometimes eyes just feel dry, scratchy, and unpleasant. Often, the meibomian glands are not functioning properly due to chronic inflammation at the level of the glands and subsequent cellular damage. There are many different avenues to pursue for treatment and symptom relief, from over-the-counter artificial tears that supplement the oily tear layer and warm compresses to prescription medications that target inflammation to light therapy.

From a dietary perspective, the goal is to decrease inflammation and oxidative stress so the glands can function better and produce more of our precious oily tear film. In a study of dry eye and Mediterranean diet intervention, there was not only an improvement in dry eye symptoms when individuals were asked about how they were feeling but also an improvement in tear film stability when objectively measured in clinic. When people adhered to a Mediterranean diet, their tears became more stable and evaporated at a slower rate. For meibomian gland dysfunction, it is the extra-virgin olive oil (EVOO) and omega fatty acids in the Mediterranean diet helping to improve function.

More dry eye research needs to be done focusing on a true Mediterranean diet as there have been many studies that do not use EVOO and instead use a lesser quality olive oil in low quantities. Thus far, it has been shown that the polyphenols contained in EVOO decrease oxidative damage and inflammation throughout the body. It could be postulated that polyphenols help decrease inflammation at the level of the meibomian glands in the eyelids just as they do in other parts of the body, though more specific research needs to be done. In addition to structural gland health, omega-3 and omega-6 fatty acids have also been shown to help increase production of meibum from the meibomian glands. Vitamin A also plays an integral role in the health of the anterior portion of the eye. Again, important sources of vitamin A are milk, yogurt, eggs, fish, tomatoes, and leafy green vegetables. All of these are common staples within the Mediterranean diet.

About Cataracts and Glaucoma

As we continue our journey toward the back of the eye, we must travel through the cornea, past the iris, through the lens and vitreous (the gel that fills the eye) where we finally arrive at the retina. Before we delve into the positive impact that the Mediterranean diet can have on retinal health, the lens deserves an honorable mention.

Humans have a clear, convex lens tucked behind the colored part of our eye, the iris. After a few decades, this lens starts to stiffen, which causes most of us to need bifocals to see at near ranges. After this, the lens can slowly become yellow and cloudy. This change in the clarity of the lens is what is known as a *cataract*. We all get cataracts if we are lucky to have enough birthdays due to the cells of the lens aging. At this time, there has not been a notable decrease in cataracts observed by adhering to a Mediterranean diet. With that said, there is currently research being done to determine if vitamin E could have therapeutic potential to push the age of cataract onset back and slow the progression of cataracts once they start. Vitamin E is abundant in leafy greens, nuts, and oregano—all components of a delicious Mediterranean salad! Even if diet ultimately does not help to influence cataract development or progression, cataract surgery is effective and now considered routine surgery.

As we continue our quest back from the lens, we arrive at the retina where the optic nerve resides. The optic nerve helps to transmit the image of what we see to our brain. Arguably the most common disease of this nerve is *glaucoma*. Glaucoma is a very common ocular disease defined by optic nerve damage, often due to elevated eye pressure. Glaucoma is typically treated with topical eye drops and microinvasive glaucoma surgeries. While the most common type of glaucoma is due to elevated eye pressure, there are other variants of the disease in which the pathophysiology is not well understood. There is ongoing research to determine to what extent inflammation may be stoking the glaucomatous fire. Depending on what this research shows, there may be a notable place for a Mediterranean diet in prevention and progression of disease.

The Retina: Macular Health, AMD, and Diabetic Retinopathy
Here we are, at the very posterior aspect of the eye—the retina. The light that enters the eye travels back to the retina. The retina then converts the image we see into an electrical signal that travels to the optic nerve and to our brain. We only utilize a small, central portion of the retina, the macula, to read and see details—think of it like a small bull's-eye responsible for detailed vision. The macula is densely pigmented and some of these pigments are supplied by our diet.

We know that the health of the macula is closely tied to three pigments—or *carotenoids*—lutein, zeaxanthin, and meso-zeaxanthin. The pigments lutein and zeaxanthin give many plants yellow or orange coloring. These pigments are provided by our diets, most commonly in the form of kale, spinach, lettuce, carrots, broccoli, and brussels sprouts. Some fruits also provide these macular pigments, though not in as substantial amounts. A few examples are avocadoes, raspberries, black currants, and nectarines. Chopping and cooking these foods with heat helps our bodies to integrate the nutrients—which sounds like a great excuse to make the savory Greek spinach pie spanakopita! Both lutein and zeaxanthin are fat-soluble, so dousing those vegetables in a splash of high-quality EVOO will help with absorption in the small intestine. Research has shown that the concentration of these carotenoids in the macula influences the concentration in the occipital cortex of the brain, where visual processing takes place. More in the macula = more in the brain.

A densely pigmented macula helps to filter and protect the eye from short-wavelength blue light. This filtering of light may help to prevent macular damage. In addition, it has been shown that these macular pigments help to improve contrast sensitivity by decreasing light scatter and glare.

Any discussion of macular health inevitably leads to age-related macular degeneration (AMD). AMD is a primary cause of blindness, affecting over 170 million people worldwide. This disease results in progressive damage to the macula in varying degrees. The understanding of the exact pathophysiology of AMD is not entirely clear, but we do know that there are many risk factors for developing the disease. Some well-established risk factors are advanced age, UV exposure, smoking, genetics, cardiovascular disease, chronic inflammation, and poor diet. While there are many contributing factors to AMD, it has been found that people with AMD have less macular pigment than those who do not. Since UV exposure is a risk factor for AMD and macular pigment helps to filter light and protect us, we want more macular pigment! The evidence for increased intake of lutein and zeaxanthin has been very well supported and dietary supplementation of these key carotenoids is widely recommended.

When we discuss dietary supplementation for AMD, it is important to note the extensive work that has been done since the late 1990s in the form of the AREDS study and the AREDS 2 study. These two very large studies focused on dietary supplementation as the means to slow progression of AMD. These studies ultimately led to the formulation of the AREDS 2 multivitamin with specific amounts of zinc, copper, vitamin E, vitamin C, lutein, and zeaxanthin. Since the development of this AREDS 2 multivitamin, there has been subsequent research focusing on AMD and the Mediterranean diet.

Before we delve into the protective effect of the Mediterranean diet further, it is important to note that the AREDS 2 multivitamin and the Mediterranean diet have not been shown to prevent AMD from occurring. A Mediterranean diet does not *explicitly* prevent us from developing early or mild AMD, despite the evidence that the dietary components are supportive of macular health. There is ongoing research about why this may be—one theory is that genetics are influencing onset of disease. Despite this, research has indeed shown that adhering to a Mediterranean diet can help to decrease risk of progression to advanced AMD.

Classification of Age-Related Macular Degeneration (AMD)	
No Macular Disease	Dietary intervention/ supplementation has <u>not</u> been shown to prevent one from developing AMD
Mild Dry AMD	**Dietary interventions shown to decrease risk of progression to advanced AMD**
Intermediate Dry AMD	
Advanced AMD *Two main types that can lead to profound vision loss and may benefit from ocular injections*	Dry – Geographic Atrophy Wet – Neovascularization

Geographic atrophy is a central lesion of the macula that leads to profound vision loss in advanced dry AMD. Geographic atrophy typically starts as a small area and then gets larger, robbing individuals of their central vision over time. There are very few pharmaceutical options for treating geographic atrophy and the ocular injections we have currently show limited benefit. A Mediterranean diet has been shown to slow enlargement of the lesion. Although it ultimately doesn't stop the geographic atrophy from getting larger long term, the lesion grows at a slower rate with the implementation of a Mediterranean diet. The current research suggests that high whole fruit and fish intake coupled with low red meat intake make an impact in this specific situation of advanced dry AMD.

Another classification of advanced AMD is neovascular or "wet" AMD, which involves irregular blood vessel growth; this condition often requires indefinite ocular injections to treat. Interestingly, a Mediterranean diet has been shown to specifically decrease risk of developing wet AMD. It is well established that a Mediterranean diet is beneficial for cardiovascular health, and it has been proposed that, for similar cellular reasons, the Mediterranean diet decreases the odds of progressing to wet AMD.

A Sidenote: Diabetic Retinopathy

Another disease that can cause unwanted, leaky retinal blood vessel growth is diabetes. Typically, ocular problems from diabetes become more prevalent the longer someone has had diabetes and the more uncontrolled their blood glucose. A Mediterranean diet enriched with nuts has been shown to decrease inflammation and lower vascular endothelial growth factor (VEGF). VEGF is a main cause of retinal neovascularization in both diabetic retinopathy and AMD. While this diet is beneficial for many reasons, it is thought to be the resveratrol found in nuts, seeds, berries, and red wine that is helping to mediate the level of unwanted VEGF in the retina.

So, while a Mediterranean diet may not decrease our risk of developing mild, early AMD (likely due to the risk factors we outlined earlier), it can decrease the speed of disease progression. Think about it in this way—one may be forced to get on the AMD train. Our diet won't change that. Life has purchased the ticket for us and the train isn't making any stops along the journey. But once we are on the train, choosing a Mediterranean diet could slow the speed of the train, so we don't reach our undesirable destination as quickly. This equates to having AMD, but also potentially having more years of functional vision and independent living.

When we think about health, there are many tools in our toolbox. One of them is our diet. What we put into our bodies matters and when it comes to our ocular health, it isn't just "eat your carrots!" Rather, it is all about balance and considering our whole selves. There is a time and a place for eye drops, for injections, for light therapy, for sunglasses, and for intentionality regarding what we eat. We are not so different than the cellular beings that came before us. We're reliant on the sun, our atmosphere, and some of the very same antioxidants, vitamins, and proteins. It is important to remember what a huge impact these building blocks can have on our vision and that means thinking hard about our diets. And when it comes to diet and ocular health, it's becoming more and more clear that the Mediterranean diet is good for our eyes. Bon appétit!

Chapter Six
The Mediterranean Table: A Prescription for Cancer Prevention and Survivorship

Shelby Terstriep, BA, MD

As an oncologist, my goal is to look at a person holistically to help treat their cancer, to decrease the chance of their cancer coming back, and to prevent other cancers and other chronic diseases. Our diet and lifestyle play a huge role in these goals. Often after a cancer diagnosis, people are very motivated to make healthy changes in their lives; I've seen people dramatically change their health for the good with food. Ultimately, my goal is to be part of a movement that seeks to improve the way we eat in the Midwest in order to prevent cancer. One such dietary movement is Midwest Mediterranean.

When we hear "Mediterranean diet," the term often creates images of sun-drenched olive groves, slower living, and lively family gatherings around a table loaded with fresh produce, olive oils, and fragrant herbs. It's easy to romanticize this lifestyle—and we should! This way of eating and living is a science-backed strategy for cancer prevention and improving survivorship outcomes. This is not only through the benefits of nutrition and obesity prevention but also from the benefits of community.

The abundance of highly processed food and the fast-paced lifestyle of the United States come at a high cost to our health and our cancer risk. According to the American Cancer Society:

- **Approximately 42 percent of all cancer cases diagnosed in the US are linked to preventable risk factors, including obesity.**
- **Obesity alone accounts for about 7–8 percent of all cancers annually, equating to roughly 85,000–100,000 preventable cases per year.**

- **Cancers with the highest attributable fractions due to obesity include:**
  - ***Endometrial cancer*: 35–50 percent of cases**
  - ***Esophageal adenocarcinoma*: ~30 percent of cases**
  - ***Postmenopausal breast cancer*: 15–20 percent of cases**
  - ***Colorectal cancer*: 11 percent of cases**
  - ***Liver and gallbladder cancer*: 50 percent of cases**

Cancer is a complex disease. At its core, cancer is a problem with cells, the tiny building blocks of our bodies. Normally, cells grow, divide, and eventually die in a very organized way. It's like a well-rehearsed dance—everything in harmony. But cancer happens when some cells go rogue. They ignore the signals telling them to stop dividing or die, and instead, they grow uncontrollably, like dandelions in a yard.

What causes this breakdown? The short answer is damaged DNA. DNA is like the instruction manual for how cells behave. When that manual gets messed up—because of genetic mutations—cells can start growing unchecked. These mutations can come from a variety of sources:

1. ***Genetics***
Some people inherit mutations from their parents that increase their cancer risk. It doesn't mean they're "destined" to get cancer, but they might have a much higher likelihood.

2. ***Environmental factors***
The world around us can damage our DNA. Ultraviolet (UV) rays from the sun, for example, can cause mutations in skin cells, leading to skin cancers. Harmful chemicals, like those in tobacco smoke or industrial pollutants, can also trigger changes in our cells. Even something as seemingly harmless as burning meat at high temperatures can release carcinogens.

3. ***Infections and inflammation***
Certain viruses and bacteria can lead to cancer. For example, human papillomavirus (HPV) can cause cervical cancer, while *Helicobacter pylori* (*H. pylori*) can contribute to stomach

cancer. Chronic inflammation—when the body's immune system is in a constant state of alert—can also damage cells over time, creating a fertile ground for cancer to develop.

4. ***Random "bad luck" mutations***
Sometimes, DNA gets damaged by sheer chance when cells divide. This is what we call "random mutations." It's no one's fault, and it's not preventable.

5. ***Lifestyle choices***
Our everyday habits play a huge role. Smoking, excessive alcohol consumption, unhealthy diets, and lack of exercise can all increase our risk.

That's a lot of "bad news." The good news is that we can take an active role in preventing cancer by creating good "Mediterranean" habits.

Targets for Lifestyle Changes
Cancers arise from a series of genetic mutations. It changes how genes are expressed and allows cells to grow uncontrollably, to escape cell death, or to spread to distant tissues—to metastasize. How can diet and lifestyle impact this complex process? To answer this question, I think about areas of risk that we can target through *lifestyle*. These include:

Oxidative stress: An imbalance between free radicals and antioxidants leads to DNA damage and mutagenesis.

Chronic inflammation: Pro-inflammatory cytokines promote tumor initiation, progression, and metastasis.

Hormonal dysregulation: Estrogen and insulin-like growth factors (IGFs) can drive cell proliferation in hormone-sensitive cancers.

Metabolic dysregulation: Obesity, insulin resistance, and hyperglycemia create an environment conducive to cancer cell survival and growth.

All of these risk areas are very common. And all of them can be partially mitigated through the most fundamental aspect of our lifestyles: *diet*.

Cancer Prevention: How the Mediterranean Diet Helps

The Mediterranean diet—rooted in whole, minimally processed foods—offers a gold-standard approach for reducing chronic disease risks, including cancer. Take these studies, for example:

> ***Breast cancer***: A landmark study published in *JAMA Internal Medicine* found that women adhering to a Mediterranean diet enriched with extra-virgin olive oil had a 62 percent lower risk of developing breast cancer.
>
> ***Colorectal cancer***: A meta-analysis in the *British Journal of Cancer* linked the Mediterranean diet with a significant reduction in colorectal cancer risk, likely due to its high fiber content.
>
> ***Survivorship***: Research in *Cancer Epidemiology, Biomarkers & Prevention* demonstrated that breast cancer survivors following a Mediterranean diet had improved survival rates and quality of life.

Rich in antioxidants, anti-inflammatory compounds, and healthy fats, this diet can help target the mechanisms that contribute to cancer's onset and spread. Let's go back to the areas of risk we outlined earlier and see how the Mediterranean diet combats each.

1. Fighting oxidative stress with antioxidants

The Mediterranean diet's emphasis on antioxidant-rich foods is central to its cancer-protective properties. Antioxidants like the ones listed below combat free radicals, reducing oxidative DNA damage, a key step in carcinogenesis.

> ***Polyphenols in olive oil***: Extra-virgin olive oil (EVOO) is rich in hydroxytyrosol and oleocanthal, especially when the oil is not filtered. These compounds have shown anti-cancer effects

in preclinical studies by inducing apoptosis in tumor cells and reducing inflammation.

Carotenoids in vegetables: Beta-carotene (carrots), lutein (spinach), and lycopene (tomatoes) scavenge free radicals and protect DNA. Lycopene, in particular, has been associated with reduced prostate cancer risk.

Flavonoids in fruits: Quercetin (apples, onions) and anthocyanins (berries) inhibit cancer cell proliferation and angiogenesis.

2. Reducing chronic inflammation

Chronic inflammation creates a microenvironment that supports tumor growth. A 2018 meta-analysis in *Nutrients* found that adherence to an anti-inflammatory diet (modeled after the Mediterranean diet) was associated with a 10–20 percent reduction in cancer risk across various types, including colorectal, breast, and gastric cancers. The Mediterranean diet reduces inflammation via multiple pathways:

Omega-3 fatty acids: In fatty fish, like salmon and sardines, omega-3s reduce pro-inflammatory eicosanoids and cytokines (e.g., IL-6, TNF-alpha).

Oleic acid in olive oil: This monounsaturated fat modulates inflammatory pathways, decreasing the expression of COX-2, a pro-inflammatory enzyme linked to tumor growth.

Herbs and spices: Turmeric (curcumin) and garlic contain bioactive compounds that suppress NF-kB, a key regulator of inflammation.

3. Balancing hormones

Hormonal imbalances can fuel cancers like breast, ovarian, and prostate. For example, the Women's Health Initiative found that dietary patterns high in plant-based foods and low in saturated fats regulated estrogen levels, correlating with lower breast cancer incidence. The Mediterranean diet supports hormone regulation in several ways:

Fiber-rich foods: Whole grains, legumes, and vegetables increase fecal excretion of estrogen, reducing circulating levels.

Plant-based phytochemicals: Isoflavones in legumes (like lentils and chickpeas) and lignans in flaxseeds are phytoestrogens that modulate estrogen activity.

Improved insulin sensitivity: High-glycemic diets can spike insulin and IGF-1, promoting cell proliferation. Mediterranean staples like whole grains, legumes, and low-sugar fruits maintain stable blood sugar levels.

4. Promoting a healthy gut microbiome

The gut microbiome plays a role in cancer prevention by modulating immune function and inflammation. Research published in *Gut* (2020) showed that Mediterranean diet adherence increased gut microbial diversity, which was associated with lower levels of inflammatory markers and a reduced risk of colorectal cancer. Fadel Nammour's chapter in our last volume of *Midwest Mediterranean* treats this issue in detail. In summary, a Mediterranean diet fosters a diverse microbiome by providing prebiotics and anti-inflammatory compounds such as:

Short-chain fatty Acids (SCFAs): Produced by gut bacteria fermenting fiber, SCFAs like butyrate suppress inflammation and enhance immune surveillance.

Polyphenols and microbiota: Polyphenols from berries, tea, and olive oil promote the growth of beneficial bacteria like *Lactobacillus* and *Bifidobacterium*.

5. Preventing and treating obesity

The Mediterranean diet focuses on nutrient-dense foods such as fruits, vegetables, whole grains, lean proteins, healthy fats, and moderate alcohol consumption. A systematic review comparing the Mediterranean diet to low-carbohydrate and low-fat diets found it to be either equally or more effective for weight reduction and improved cardiovascular risk factors, making it a preferred choice for obesity treatment.

The superior performance of this diet for preventing and treating obesity in the studies is likely due to a variety of things. First, the Mediterranean way of eating is more palatable and not as restrictive as other "diet plans" and therefore is easier to follow over the long term. Second, a study found that individuals following the Mediterranean diet exhibited more stable levels of appetite-regulating hormones compared to those on Western diets. Leptin is one of those hormones. It is secreted by our fat glands and tells our brains that we are full. People having trouble losing weight often have leptin resistance where the brain isn't recognizing this signal. Increasing fiber and eating low-processed foods are two ways to help treat leptin resistance.

The Mediterranean diet is also helpful in reducing abdominal obesity, which is particularly harmful due to its association with metabolic syndrome and inflammation. A study in individuals with metabolic syndrome showed that the Mediterranean diet reduced the fat around our organs, independent of total body weight changes, improving insulin sensitivity and reducing systemic inflammation, which can also help regulate leptin.

All of these factors are extremely helpful for both cancer prevention and reducing risk of cancer recurrence.

Cancer Survivorship:
The Mediterranean Diet's Role in Recovery

For cancer survivors, the journey doesn't end with remission. After a successful battle with cancer, the goal shifts from surviving to reducing recurrence risk, to reducing the risk of a second cancer, and to improving overall well-being. Here's where the Mediterranean diet shines:

1. ***Weight management and insulin sensitivity***
   Obesity and insulin resistance are linked to higher recurrence rates in cancers like breast and colorectal. The Mediterranean diet's emphasis on whole, nutrient-dense

foods aids in maintaining a healthy weight and improving insulin sensitivity.

2. ***Enhancing energy levels during treatment***
Cancer treatments like chemotherapy and radiation can be taxing. The Mediterranean diet provides an energy-rich yet balanced approach, with complex carbohydrates, lean proteins, and healthy fats to fuel the body without overwhelming it.

3. ***Supporting cardiovascular health***
Many cancer survivors face increased cardiovascular risks due to treatment side effects. Foods like nuts, seeds, and olive oil support heart health, reducing the long-term risks for survivors.

4. ***Mitigating treatment side effects***
Nausea, loss of appetite, and altered taste buds are common challenges. Incorporating small, flavorful Mediterranean-inspired meals—like an herbed hummus with fresh vegetables or a comforting lentil soup—can make eating more enjoyable and nutritious during these times.

Impact of Social Support on Cancer Prevention and Survivorship

One of the hallmarks of the Mediterranean lifestyle is the tradition of communal meals, which foster social connection and emotional support. A study on Mediterranean dietary patterns found that frequent communal eating was associated with lower levels of depression and anxiety. Sharing meals strengthens relationships, which in turn contributes to mental health. This emphasis on connection complements the physical and nutritional aspects of the Mediterranean diet. Scientific studies underline how social support, a key element of the Mediterranean lifestyle, contributes to improved health outcomes, including reduced risks of cancer and improved quality of life.

Social support and connection can even influence many factors associated with cancer outcomes including:

- **Reduction of cortisol levels, which, when elevated chronically, can suppress the immune system and promote tumor growth.**
- **Likelihood to engage in physical activity, maintain a healthy diet, and avoid smoking.**
- **Likelihood to follow the recommended cancer screening guidelines, such as mammograms or colonoscopies, leading to earlier detection and better outcomes.**
- **Better mental and physical health outcomes, including improved survival rates. A large meta-analysis found that cancer patients with strong social support had a 50 percent higher likelihood of survival compared to those with limited social ties. Social support was particularly impactful for breast, colorectal, and lung cancer.**

Community and social connection play a vital role in cancer prevention and survivorship. By fostering healthy behaviors, reducing stress, enhancing immune function, and promoting emotional resilience, strong social ties can significantly improve outcomes. Leveraging social support through family, friends, support groups, and community engagement should be a key part of cancer care strategies.

Practical Tips for People

As physicians, we often talk about "what to do." The "how to do it" is just as important. Here's how I guide my patients to adopt Mediterranean principles:

> ***Start small***: For example, replace one processed snack with a handful of almonds or fresh fruit. Develop your own protocol of how you want to eat that includes the principles of Mediterranean eating and slowly make the changes until you are at that goal. For example, one aspect of my protocol is that I have six fruits and vegetables per day. Every morning I eat fruit. Lunch and dinner include two servings of vegetables, and I have a snack with fruit in it. I don't have to think about how I'm getting my fiber in that way.

Experiment with herbs and spices: Flavor meals with anti-inflammatory ingredients like turmeric, garlic, and rosemary. Use those seasonings to help flavor your olive oil too! This is awesome for drizzling on vegetables that you roast or for making your own homemade dressings.

Build balanced plates: Aim for half your plate as vegetables, a quarter as lean protein (like fish or legumes), and a quarter as whole grains.

Go local, go seasonal: Midwestern farmers markets offer fresh produce like squash, tomatoes, and berries, all staples of Mediterranean cuisine.

Romanticize your life: Slow down, take it all in, find joy in the little things each day. Light the candles at the dinner table and eat with intention.

Group meals: Regularly share meals with family and friends to foster connection. Meet friends for lunch. Have Sunday night dinners where everyone brings a dish. Put the phone down during meals.

The Bottom Line

The Mediterranean diet is more than just a way of eating—it's a lifestyle and a powerful tool in cancer prevention and survivorship and we can partake of it right here in the Midwest. Midwest Mediterranean is about filling your plate with real foods that heal, energize, and support the body's natural defenses, and it's also about the connection that sharing a good meal with others provides.

Whether you're trying to reduce your cancer risk, are a survivor working to rebuild strength, or are simply someone aiming for a healthier lifestyle, this diet offers a delicious, sustainable, and scientifically backed path forward.

This is the prescription I wish every person could receive: Eat abundantly, eat joyfully, and let food be a cornerstone of healing.

Chapter Seven
Socrates Visits the Doctor: The Mediterranean Diet and Quality of Life

Mark Rostad, MD

What makes life worth living? Socrates seemed to address this when he said, "The unexamined life is not worth living." Assuming Socrates actually said this, as Plato claims in *The Apology*, we can assume that the great Athenian philosopher thought that the examined life is worth living. At the risk of blaspheming one of the greatest minds in human history, I must disagree with Socrates. Before you throw this book in the trash and call me an arrogant moron, I don't wholly disagree with the man considered by many to be the father of Western philosophy. I would simply rephrase his statement to read: "The unexamined life *may* not be worth living."

In his 1942 essay, *The Myth of Sisyphus*, French philosopher Albert Camus wrote, "Deciding whether or not life is worth living is to answer the fundamental question in philosophy." If this is true, then I doubt that humanity will ever establish a definitive answer. This is why I would like to amend Socrates's statement. It is not his sentiment that I take issue with, but rather the assuredness of his language.

In specifically addressing ideas from two of history's great philosophers, I am hoping to make clear the inherent individuality and, therefore, ambiguity in the question "What makes life worth living?" If Albert Camus is correct and this question strikes at the heart of philosophy itself, the breadth of answers could range from "nothing" to "everything" to "42." It is precisely this seemingly infinite variation that led me to choose a career in healthcare that revolves around the concept of quality of life.

I am a palliative care physician. For those unfamiliar with this medical subspecialty, I care for patients who live with serious, typically incurable, illness. The patients whom I most commonly see are those who suffer from metastatic cancer. The term metastatic refers to when a cancer has spread from its place of origin to other areas of the body. An example of this would be when pancreatic cancer travels from the pancreas to the liver or lungs, attaches to those organs, and then begins to grow. When cancer of one organ spreads to another, it is often thought to be incurable. However, incurable does not mean untreatable.

An incurable disease is a pathology that can be managed or "held at bay" through medical therapies but will never be entirely eradicated. The classic examples are diseases like dementia, Parkinson's disease, amyotrophic lateral sclerosis (ALS), and many metastatic cancers. Chronic obstructive pulmonary disease (COPD), heart failure, liver cirrhosis, and chronic kidney disease are also considered incurable diseases with the exception of patients who are well enough and young enough to receive an organ transplant. These incurable illnesses are very different than untreatable diseases—defined as illnesses for which there are no medical options by which to extend life. An untreatable disease is best addressed with hospice care. An incurable disease, on the other hand, is managed by a palliative care clinician, like me.

I often describe living with an incurable disease like sharing a home with someone who routinely breaks things, never fixes anything, never buys anything, eats all the food in the fridge, never cooks, never shares, never stops talking, and never leaves. To make matters worse, this metaphorical roommate follows you to work, to the grocery store, to the gym, and even to the restroom. People suffering from incurable illness have every aspect of their life affected. So, if we can't cure the disease, or "evict the roommate," how can we help improve the person's quality of life? Since each of us has control over what we eat, one high impact point to improve quality of life is *diet*. Of the seemingly countless different diet options, the Mediterranean diet has by far the best evidence to support its impact on overall quality of life.

But if quality of life is directly related to the question of "what makes life worth living," how can we measure this quality with any semblance of objectivity? Numerous researchers have tried to answer this. There are different tools that have been developed to try and quantify health-related quality of life. Three such tools are the SF-12, SF-20, and SF-36 Health Surveys. These surveys were originally developed by RAND, a nonprofit, nonpartisan research organization known for their Medical Outcomes Study (MOS). There have been many other tools published over the years—the Manchester Short Assessment of Quality of Life (MANSA) and the EuroQol 5-Dimension: Health-Related Quality of Life (EQ-5D) questionnaire are two examples. Unfortunately, the fact that quality of life is such a nuanced and complicated topic means there is no universally accepted method of measurement. I'm mentioning all this because the ambiguity inherent in our topic must be kept in mind as we explore the literature investigating "quality of life" and the Mediterranean diet.

What does the literature say?

In 2015, a team of Dutch researchers considered the idea that dietary patterns could impact healthy life expectancy, which is defined as the duration of life lived in good health and free of disease. They measured quality-adjusted life years in people with three different eating patterns—the World Health Organization's guidelines for a healthy diet, the Dutch guidelines for a healthy diet, and the Mediterranean diet. The team put together an algorithm to rate adherence over time to these respective diets. They had a cohort of over thirty-three thousand participants and monitored patients for roughly fifteen years. The group was observed for the development of diseases including cancer, arthritis, various heart diseases, diabetes, stroke, and COPD. If these ailments occurred, it was factored into the calculation of the person's quality-adjusted life years. This was measured on a scale of 0 to 1 where 0 was death and 1 was perfect health; the more disease a patient had, the lower their number would be in terms of quality-adjusted life years. What the Dutch team ultimately found was that of the three predefined diets, those with the greatest level of adherence to the Mediterranean diet had the greatest number of quality-adjusted life years. In other words, the people who stuck to the Mediterranean diet lived with less disease and for longer compared to those who ate other diets.

This same group of researchers also published a separate study using roughly the same cohort that calculated disability-adjusted life years (DALYs) rather than quality-adjusted life years (QALYs). What is the difference between these measurements? DALYs help to understand disease burden in a population whereas QALYs help identify the benefit of particular interventions on extending healthy life. Simply put, DALYs are the number of healthy years lost while QALYs are the number of healthy years gained.

When exploring disability-adjusted life years, the Dutch team of researchers used different metrics. Rather than looking at three different predefined diets, they developed a composite score related to four different lifestyle factors–smoking, BMI, exercise, and adherence to the Mediterranean diet. What the team found was that people with lower composite scores (i.e., those who smoked, were overweight according to BMI, did not exercise, and did not follow the Mediterranean diet) had roughly -2 DALYs. This means that the non-smokers from the study who had a BMI < 25, exercised regularly, and adhered to a Mediterranean diet lived about two years longer in good health.

Further evidence supporting the impact of the Mediterranean diet on quality of life comes from an investigation into osteoarthritis. Arthritis simply means inflammation of one or more joints. Osteoarthritis is the type of "wear-and-tear" arthritis that every human being will experience if they live long enough. It is entirely different than rheumatoid arthritis, which is caused by a person's own immune system misbehaving and attacking one's own joints. Regardless of the cause of joint inflammation, the impact arthritis can have on quality of life can be profound. It can lead to pain, decreased mobility, decreased strength, decreased socialization, increased loneliness, and depression.

Knowing this, a group of Italian and British researchers sought to investigate the impact of the Mediterranean diet on quality of life among patients with osteoarthritis. They utilized the roughly 4,800 patient dataset from the Osteoarthritis Initiative (OAI), which was a large, ten-year North American study conducted to better understand osteoarthritis in order to improve methods of prevention and treatment. What they found was a consistent improvement in quality of life in relation to the degree of adherence to the Mediterranean diet. The researchers were able to break this down further and found that the study participants most adherent to the Mediterranean diet had less joint pain, better mobility, and less depression. Learning this, it is no wonder why the study clearly demonstrated a connection between improved quality of life and the Mediterranean diet.

Two more studies that further support the Mediterranean diet's use to improve quality of life come from the journal *Experimental Gerontology* in 2023. One investigation, called the PREDIDEP study, was out of Spain. It was a two-year multicenter, randomized, single-blinded trial. This study explored whether a Mediterranean diet improved quality of life among patients with depression. What they found were distinct improvements in both the study participants' mental health and perceived vitality. To put this more bluntly, the people who followed the Mediterranean diet had better mood, more energy, and less depression. (William Schultz's chapter in volume one of this series treats this issue in more detail.)

The other study from *Experimental Gerontology* was another Italian investigation. It explored the Mediterranean diet's effect on quality of life and overall cognition. This study was specifically focused on older adults rather than adults with a history of dementia, as was the case in the Spanish trial I just mentioned. This caveat particularly caught my eye as the World Health Organization estimates that the population of people over sixty will increase from one billion in 2020 to two billion in 2050. With increased age comes an increased likelihood of cognitive decline. According to the 2019 Global Burden of Diseases, Injuries, and Risk Factors Study (GBD) from the Dementia Forecasting Collaborators, the estimated number of people suffering with dementia will climb to around 153 million in 2050. Could adherence to the Mediterranean diet help maintain or even improve cognition in people over sixty? This Italian study seems to answer, "Yes."

Digging into the meat of the study, the investigators found that those with the highest adherence to the Mediterranean diet had distinctly less cognitive impairment compared to those who did not adhere to the diet. Even more intriguing, implementing the Mediterranean diet seemed to help stave off dementia even when the results were adjusted to account for differences in sex, age, education, occupation, smoking habits, and physical activity. Other benefits of high adherence to the Mediterranean diet identified in this 2023 Italian study included better sleep, less depression, and improved quality of life.

As a palliative care physician, I am always considering ways to improve quality of life. To accomplish this, I start every patient visit by exploring the patient's definition of "What makes life worth living?" In doing so, I hear a wide variety of answers. Examples of things I commonly hear are:

> "Talking with my wife."
> "Playing with my grandkids."
> "Joking with my family."
> "Playing the piano."
> "Driving my car."
> "Hiking in the woods."
> "Enjoying meals with friends."

For patients who consider any of these examples to add quality to their lives, I recommend the Mediterranean diet. To put it plainly, if a patient finds joy in conversation with loved ones or being physically independent and mobile, the Mediterranean diet will help maintain these crucial aspects of life. I believe Socrates would consider the preservation of these qualities as demonstration of a well-examined life.

Conclusion
Final Thoughts at the Table . . .

Megan Myrdal and Peter Schultz

As we conclude *Midwest Mediterranean* 2.0, we hope you'll share our opinion that this diet—or lifestyle, as we should really call it—is truly something exceptional. By bringing together healthy, sustainably grown foods of the upper Midwest with the key ingredients, flavors, and techniques of the Mediterranean, along with the knowledge of this diet's history, an appreciation for the food of our region, and medical knowledge—we feel that this little book is truly something unique and special.

However, reading can only get you so far.

In order to understand how truly awesome this idea is, *you really must taste it*.

That's why we conclude this book with a collection of amazing recipes from chefs and home cooks from across the Midwest *and* the Mediterranean. The folks who shared these recipes are truly the best of the best. Not only do they cook it, but they live it too! You will see ingredients and techniques that are familiar, and others that may be new. You'll see high-quality ingredients from Midwest farmers, like beans and oats, and high-quality ingredients from Mediterranean farmers, like extra-virgin olive oil from Mistra Estates. These recommendations are key! In the famous words of Alice Waters, "When you have the best and tastiest ingredients, you can cook very simply, and the food will be extraordinary, because it tastes like what it is."

We're blessed to have some of the best and tastiest ingredients right in our backyard, and some brought to us from our friends across the world, to create extraordinary Midwest Mediterranean food.

Finally, as we developed this little book of Midwest Mediterranean principles and particulars, the most thrilling part was the idea of the "eclectic community table" that we hope you and your friends and family will create. As you develop your own delicious table using these foods and ideas, we hope you will share it with others and let them discover this truly amazing way of eating and living.

Bon appétit!

Appendix A

More Mediterranean Recipes for the High Plains

1. **Spinach and Artichoke Dip Twice-Baked Potatoes** | Heather Schneider
2. **Grilled Salmon and Orzo Salad** | William DeHoogh
3. **French Onion Soup . . . my way!** | Niki Cutler-Shea
4. **Spicy Midwest Mediterranean Chicken and Vegetables** | Antonio Hinojosa
5. **Basil and Pistachio Pesto** | Kirsten Theye
6. **Greek Almond Cookies** | Susan Mathison
7. **Spanakopita** | Cameron Tibbits
8. **Rustic Tomato Tart** | Kim Bailey
9. **Plate Licker Butternut Squash** | Ron and Amanda Phillips
10. **Lambriano** | Aspasia Stamataki
11. **Midwest Mediterranean Ranch** | Megan Myrdal
12. **The Ultimate Mediterranean Chicken and Rice** | Peter Schultz
13. **Fennel A.F.** | Sarah Fisher
14. **Greek Island Fish Salad** | Sam Wai
15. **Rustic Tomato Basil Soup** | Julie Garden-Robinson
16. **Winter Grain Bowl** | Cady Ann Rutter

Spinach and Artichoke Dip Twice-Baked Potatoes

Heather Schneider

A Midwest classic with a Mediterranean twist!

Yield ~ 4 servings
Active time ~ 30 minutes
Total time ~ 60 minutes

Ingredients

- 4 North Dakota-grown potatoes
- Extra-virgin olive oil
- ½ cup (115g) cottage cheese
- ½ cup (115g) Greek yogurt
- ¼ cup (25g) parmesan cheese
- 1 small shallot, minced
- 1 small garlic clove, minced
- ½ tsp onion powder
- ½ tsp oregano
- ½ tsp rosemary
- Salt and black pepper
- 1 cup (6 ounces) shredded mozzarella cheese
- 2 cups (4 ounces) raw baby spinach, chopped
- 8 ounces (225g) canned artichokes, drained and chopped
- Zest and juice of one lemon

Crispy Topping *(optional)*

- 1 cup shredded parmesan cheese
- 3 tbsp melted butter
- ½ tsp thyme
- ½ tsp basil

- Salt and pepper
- 1 cup panko breadcrumbs
- 2 tbsp fresh parsley, chopped, to garnish

Directions

1. If using only the oven: Preheat oven to 375°F (190°C). Using a fork or paring knife, puncture potatoes in several spots. Rub each potato with a light coat of olive oil. Arrange on a rack set on a baking sheet, or directly on an oven rack, and bake until a fork can easily be inserted into the center of each potato, about 1 hour. If setting potatoes directly on oven rack, set a sheet of foil on the rack below to catch any oil drips.
2. If using the microwave and oven: Preheat oven to 450°F (230°C). Using a fork or paring knife, puncture potatoes in several spots. Microwave potatoes for 5 minutes. Rub each potato with a light coat of olive oil. Arrange on a rack set on a baking sheet, or directly on an oven rack, and bake until a fork can easily be inserted into the center of each potato, about 20 minutes. If setting potatoes directly on oven rack, set a sheet of foil on the rack below to catch any oil drips.
3. Let potatoes rest 5 minutes.
4. Meanwhile, in a large mixing bowl, stir together yogurt, cottage cheese, parmesan cheese, shallot, garlic, seasonings, salt, and pepper.
5. Slice each potato open lengthwise and carefully scoop flesh into the mixing bowl with the other ingredients.
6. Mash the potatoes with a fork while mixing with the other ingredients, then fold in mozzarella cheese, artichokes, spinach, and lemon. Scoop potato mixture back into the baked potato skins and shape back into the classic baked potato shape.
7. Top with a generous amount of panko/parmesan topping and drizzle with olive oil.
8. Return to a 375° oven and cook until the cheese has melted and begun to brown in spots, about 15–20 minutes. Serve warm and garnish with fresh chopped parsley.

Grilled Salmon and Orzo Salad

William DeHoogh

This dish is the perfect match for a hot summer's day and fresh produce from the garden. Consider this recipe to be a starting point that can be endlessly adapted. The grilled salmon can be swapped with smoked salmon, roast chicken, or grilled shrimp. Israeli couscous or farro can be substituted for orzo. Other fresh vegetables from the garden, such as zucchini or eggplant, can also be grilled and added to the salad.

Yield ~ 4 servings
Prep Time ~ 15 minutes
Total Time ~ 45 minutes

Ingredients

Dressing

- ¼ cup extra-virgin olive oil
- 1 ½ tbsp white wine vinegar or champagne vinegar
- ½ tbsp lemon juice
- ½ shallot, finely minced
- 2 tsp miso paste or Dijon mustard
- 1 clove garlic, minced
- Salmon
- 4 skin-on salmon fillets (4 ounces each)
- Kosher salt and black pepper

Salad

- 8 ounces orzo or Israeli couscous, cooked according to package directions
- 4 ounces fresh mozzarella cheese, torn into small pieces
- ½ medium cucumber, peeled, seeded, and sliced into half moons
- 6 ounces cherry tomatoes, halved

- 1 tbsp fresh basil leaves, or other fresh herbs such as parsley or mint, roughly chopped
- 2 tsp lemon zest

Directions

1. Preheat the grill to medium-high heat.
2. Combine the dressing ingredients in a small bowl, whisking until fully emulsified.
3. Cook orzo in salted water according to package directions, drain, toss with a drizzle of olive oil, and set aside to cool.
4. Season salmon with kosher salt and black pepper (or your favorite seafood seasoning mix) and grill skin side down until salmon is opaque. Using an instant-read thermometer, remove from heat once it reaches an internal temp of 130 degrees, about 8–10 minutes total. Remove and discard salmon skin. Set salmon fillets aside while you finish assembling the salad.
5. Assemble the salad in a large bowl by combining the orzo, mozzarella, cucumber, tomatoes, and lemon zest until evenly distributed. Recombine dressing and mix into salad. Season to taste with kosher salt and black pepper.
6. Divide salad among 4 plates and top with the salmon fillets. Optionally, garnish with additional herbs and lemon zest

French Onion Soup . . . My Way!

Niki Cutler-Shea

Another Mediterranean classic transformed into an every week American staple!

Yield ~ 5–6 servings
Prep Time ~ 15 minutes
Total Time ~ 45 minutes

Ingredients

- 4 tbsp unsalted butter
- 5 large sweet onions, halved and thinly sliced
- 1 tsp salt
- 2 spoonfuls minced garlic
- 1 cup red wine
- 32 ounces low-sodium beef broth
- 24 ounces low-sodium chicken broth
- 2 tbsp Worcestershire sauce
- Fresh thyme, or dried, to taste
- 2 bay leaves
- 1 tbsp balsamic vinegar
- Salt and pepper, to taste
- 1 ½ cups shredded Gruyère
- ¼ cup shredded mozzarella
- Handful of shredded Parmesan

Directions

1. In a large pot combine butter, sliced onions, and garlic over medium-high heat. Sauté, stirring frequently until the onions are soft.
2. Reduce to medium heat and add in salt and sugar. Cook for about

30–40 minutes, stirring every few minutes until caramelized.

3. Add red wine, broths, Worcestershire, thyme, bay leaves, and vinegar. Lower heat and simmer for around 20 minutes.
4. Here's where I change things up: I ladle the soup into bowls and top with the 3 cheeses, but I don't top the soup with toasted French bread and I don't bake in the oven to melt the cheese.
5. Instead, I serve the bread on the side, topping French bread slices with a layer of bechamel sauce, then shredded Gruyère, and bake until golden brown, about 10 minutes at 350°F.

Add a simple green salad and you've got yourself an amazing lunch or dinner!

Spicy Midwest Mediterranean Chicken and Vegetables

Antonio Hinojosa

This guy knows spices!

Yield ~ 4 servings
Prep Time ~ 20 minutes
Total Time ~ 50 minutes

Ingredients

- 1–2 lbs chicken breast or thighs, cut into bite-size pieces
- 4 tbsp liquid gold (aka Mistra Estates extra-virgin olive oil)
- 2 tbsp unsalted butter
- 3 tbsp Hinospice #2 or #3 (the more you add, the spicier and more flavorful
- without the salt)
- 1 tsp cracked peppercorn
- 4 ounces sauvignon blanc wine (may substitute with any broth of your choosing)
- ½ tbsp red chili flakes (or more, to taste)
- 1 tbsp coarse sea salt
- 1 tbsp coarse black pepper
- 1 tsp cumin
- 2 fresh garlic cloves, finely chopped
- 1 tsp Italian seasoning
- 3 medium green onions, sliced and divided (use greens for garnish)
- 1 bunch of asparagus (~10 ounces), cut into 4 pieces per stalk
- 2 fresh jalapeños, thinly sliced

To serve: Cooked orzo or wild rice

Directions

1. In a container or zip-top bag, add the chicken and 2 tbsp of liquid gold, cracked black pepper, and 2 tbsp of Hinospice.
2. Marinate for at least 2 hours or up to 4 hours in the refrigerator, turning and mixing every 30–40 minutes. The longer you marinate, the better.
3. Next, heat 1 tbsp oil and 1 tbsp butter in a non-stick skillet.
4. Once the oil and butter mixture are hot, add the chicken and cook for 3–4 minutes, continuously stirring.
5. Remove the chicken from the skillet and add the remainder of the oil and butter. Add the vegetables along with the rest of the seasonings. Cook for 1–2 minutes, then add chicken with its juices back to the pan and continue to cook for 2–3 minutes.
6. Deglaze the pan with the wine and a pat of butter.
7. Serve on top of a mound of seasoned orzo or wild rice. Season with salt and pepper to taste.
8. Garnish with tomato slices, sliced green onion, and a drizzle of liquid gold.

   Note: If you aren't using a non-stick skillet, dust the chicken in flour to prevent sticking.

Basil and Pistachio Pesto

Kirsten Theye

I'm not sure exactly when our love affair with pesto began, but we are now at the point where we nurture almost one hundred basil plants in our backyard every summer so that we can make enough pesto to last all year. We use our pesto as a sauce for pasta, bruschetta, pizza, and panini—or we just add a spoonful to tomato soup or fettuccine alfredo. I use pistachios instead of pine nuts because their mild creaminess offsets some of the bitterness from the basil leaves—plus they add to the vibrant green of the pesto. This is a proportional recipe, based on how much fresh basil you have, so you can make just a little for an appetizer or several jars worth to store in the freezer.

PREP TIME ~ 5 to 45 minutes, depending on how much basil you have to de-stem
TOTAL TIME ~ 10 to 50 minutes

Ingredients

- Fresh basil
- Parmesan (either torn into 1-inch chunks or shredded)
- Pistachios
- Garlic cloves
- Salt and black pepper
- High-quality olive oil

Directions

1. Remove tough stems from the ends of your basil leaves and then weigh your basil in grams. Be sure to note this number!
2. Wash the basil leaves well and then spin or pat them dry.
3. Time to do a non-threatening amount of math! Divide the number of grams of basil into two. (The goal is to use about half as many grams of parmesan and pistachios as you have basil. For example, if you have 100g of basil, you'll want about 50g of parmesan and 50g of pistachios.)

4. In a food processor, add the weighed parmesan and pistachios, 2 cloves of garlic per 100g of basil, and salt and pepper.
5. Grind up the mixture and then add the basil. Drizzle in olive oil as it spins, stopping periodically to scrape the sides and enjoy the smell of summer. Once all of the basil is incorporated, taste it! I invariably find that it needs more salt.

Notes

This recipe is abundantly flexible so it's okay if you weigh your ingredients with your heart instead of your kitchen scale. I use much less basil earlier in the summer when my plants are still tiny and more later on when the basil is plentiful.

If I'm serving this pesto in its fresh state to more sensitive groups, I sauté the garlic cloves for a few minutes first to take out the harsh bite. If I'm serving it cooked (like on a pizza), I don't worry about it because the garlic will mellow in the oven.

If I'm making the pesto to freeze, or for pizza, I add just enough olive oil for the pesto to be able to spin in the food processor. If I'm making the pesto to serve on pasta, I add a bit more.

Whether I store it in the fridge or the freezer, I pour a thin layer of olive oil on the top.

Greek Almond Cookies

Susan Mathison

Tasty, super easy—and not too sweet! The absolute heart of the Mediterranean diet is keeping your sugar modest. We don't need to give it up altogether, but moderation will be our best medicine!

Yield ~ about 24 medium-sized cookies
Prep Time ~ 15 minutes
Total Time ~ 45 minutes

Ingredients

- 3 cups finely ground blanched almond flour
- 1 cup sweetener—monkfruit/allulose blend
- 3 whipped egg whites (to soft peaks)
- 1 tsp vanilla extract
- ½ tsp almond extract
- ¼ cup fresh lemon juice
- 1 tbsp lemon zest
- Toasted sliced almonds, to top

Directions

1. Preheat your oven to 350°F and line a baking sheet with parchment paper.
2. In a large mixing bowl, combine 3 cups of finely ground blanched almond flour and 1 cup of sweetener. Mix well to combine.
3. In a separate mixing bowl, whip 3 egg whites to soft peaks. An electric mixer or beater is fine if you don't want to hand whip.
4. Add 1 tsp of vanilla extract and ½ tsp of almond extract to the egg whites and continue whipping gently.
5. Gradually fold the whipped egg whites into the almond flour mixture, being careful not to overmix.

6. Add ¼ cup of fresh lemon juice and 1 tbsp of lemon zest to the mixture and continue to fold until well combined. The dough will be a bit sticky.
7. Form the dough into small balls (about the size of a golf ball) and place them on the lined baking sheet. Press some sliced almonds into the top of each ball.
8. Press down with the palm of your hand to flatten into circles, but don't make them too thin.
9. Bake for 15–20 minutes, or until the cookies are light golden brown.
10. Leave cookies on the pan until cool, as they are fragile.

Notes

These would be considered gluten-free, low-carb, and keto-friendly.

You could replace part of the almond flour with almond meal, if you'd like a bit more texture to the dough.

The monk fruit/allulose blend works well because you can measure it 1:1 as a sugar substitute. Monk fruit is a bit sweeter than cane or sugar beet sugar, while allulose is less sweet, so the combination works well. It tastes, bakes, browns, and dissolves just like sugar. There are many brands available online, and I've been able to find it at some of my local grocery stores.

SPANAKOPITA

Cameron Tibbits

This is a Greek classic transformed for ease and taste by a genius from Texas.

YIELD ~ 8 servings
PREP TIME ~ 15 minutes
TOTAL TIME ~ 55 minutes

INGREDIENTS

- ½ large white onion, diced
- 16 ounces fresh baby spinach
- 2 ounces dry white wine
- ¾ -ounce container fresh dill, finely chopped
- 6–8 large fresh mint leaves, finely chopped
- 1 tbsp fresh oregano, finely chopped
- 1 egg
- 7-ounce block of feta cheese, crumbled
- 2 pie crusts
- Greek salt
- ¼ cup Mistra Estates extra-virgin olive oil
- Fresh ground pepper, to taste.

DIRECTIONS

1. Preheat oven to 375°F.
2. In a very large pot, sauté the onion in olive oil on medium-high until translucent (about 5 minutes). Lower heat to medium.
3. Add the spinach, a touch of salt, and wine. Cover and cook, mixing occasionally until almost completely wilted.
4. Meanwhile, add the feta and egg to a medium mixing bowl and mix well.
5. Add the herbs to the spinach and cook uncovered an additional 2–3

mins until the spinach is completely wilted. Pour spinach mixture into a fine metal sieve and push with a spatula to remove as much moisture as possible.

6. Place the spinach onto a cutting board and roughly chop the mixture. If there is a lot of water on the board, you will need to squeeze more water from the spinach.
7. Add the chopped spinach to the bowl with the feta and egg mixture and combine with a touch more salt and a generous grind of fresh black pepper.
8. Oil a piece of parchment paper on a baking sheet. Lay 1 pie crust on the parchment paper and add the spinach and feta mixture, spreading it out from the middle. Leave about 2 inches at the edge. Place a very light coating of olive oil on the edge to help seal with the top crust.
9. Place the second pie crust on top and press down around the edges. Using your thumb and index finger, go around the circle folding up to insure a good seal.
10. Brush with olive oil and bake on the middle oven rack for 35 minutes, or until golden brown.
11. Remove and rest for 5 minutes before cutting.

Rustic Tomato Tart

Kim Bailey

This little gem is adapted from Sarah Nasello and The Pioneer Woman.

YIELD ~ 8 servings
PREP TIME ~ 15 minutes
TOTAL TIME ~ 40–45 minutes

Ingredients

- 1 - 9–10" pie crust, uncooked
- 1 large red onion, thinly sliced
- 2 tbsp butter
- 1 tbsp extra-virgin olive oil
- ½ tsp salt
- ½ tsp pepper
- 1 cup grated cheese (a mixture of parmesan, Gruyère, and fontina, or just cheddar)
- 1 pint cherry or grape tomatoes, or 3 large heirloom tomatoes, sliced ¼" to ½" thick
- Salt & pepper to taste
- Handful of fresh basil, thinly sliced

Directions

1. Place pie crust on a rimmed baking sheet or round pizza pan. Set aside.
2. In a large skillet, heat butter and oil over medium heat. Add sliced onion, season with salt and pepper, and cook for 20–25 minutes, stirring occasionally until the onions are soft and caramelized to a light brown color.
3. Slice heirloom tomatoes in thick slices and let drain on a paper towel for a few minutes.

4. Leaving a 1-inch border on the crust, sprinkle cheese, layer with onions, and top with tomatoes. Add a pinch of salt and pepper. Fold edges of the crust up over the edge of tomato mixture. If desired, brush with a mixture of beaten egg and milk.
5. Bake at 425°F for 10 minutes. Turn the oven down to 375° to finish baking, approximately 10–15 more minutes. Top with sliced fresh basil, and serve in wedges, warm or at room temperature.

PLATE LICKER BUTTERNUT SQUASH

Ron and Amanda Phillips

The name says it all!

YIELD ~ 5–6 servings
PREP TIME ~ 15 minutes
TOTAL TIME ~ 60 minutes

INGREDIENTS

- 3 strips of bacon
- 1 medium butternut squash, peeled and cut into 1-inch cubes
- 1 bag of brussels sprouts (~ 20 ounces, stemmed and cut in half
- 1 cup dried cranberries or dried cherries
- 1 package of crumbled feta cheese (6–8 ounces)
- Mistra Estates extra-virgin olive oil
- Salt
- Pepper
- Greek seasonings
- Reduced balsamic vinegar

DIRECTIONS

1. Preheat oven to 350°F.
2. Add 3 strips of bacon to a large sheet pan and start cooking.
3. In a large bowl, mix together the butternut squash, brussels sprouts, a generous amount of Mistra Estates extra-virgin olive oil, salt, pepper, and Greek seasoning.
4. When the bacon is about half-cooked, remove from the sheet and break into pieces. Add to the veggie mixture and mix well. Spread everything evenly on the sheet pan and pop back in the oven for about 45 minutes.

5. Sprinkle half of the package of crumbled feta and a cup of cranberries on top of the veggies. Bake for another 15 minutes, or until fork tender.
6. Remove and sprinkle the rest of the feta on top.
7. Drizzle with balsamic vinegar, then devour the deliciousness!

LAMBRIANO

Aspasia Stamataki

This is a traditional dish for Easter from the mountainous Cretan village of Kapetaniana.

YIELD ~ 6–8 servings
PREP TIME ~ 15 minutes
TOTAL TIME ~ 120 minutes

INGREDIENTS

- 2 kilos lamb
- 3 cups rice
- 7 cups water
- 250g full fat yogurt
- 200g sour cream
- Salt and pepper

DIRECTIONS

1. Place the rice in a pot with the seasoned lamb on top.
2. Pour the yogurt and the sour cream on top of the lamb and add the water.
3. Bake in the oven at 200°C for 2 hours. (Cover the pot in the beginning and leave it open toward the end to give the meat a nice color.)

Midwest Mediterranean Ranch

Megan Myrdal

You'll find many variations of homemade ranch dressing on the internet and in cookbooks. I've adapted this recipe over time to meet my desire for a tangy, flavorful ranch, while still being familiar and enjoyable to the kids. It's a personal family favorite. I like to use nonfat Greek yogurt and buttermilk to keep calories down and add a little protein, and to add the fat from extra-virgin olive oil. Of all the forms of fat, extra-virgin olive oil has the most scientific evidence to support its use for heart and overall health. And it's delicious!

Yield ~ 1 ½ cups
Serving Size ~ 2 tbsp
Prep Time ~ 15 minutes

Ingredients

- 1 cup nonfat Greek yogurt
- 1 tsp garlic powder
- ½ tsp dill weed
- ½ tsp onion powder
- ½ tsp parsley
- 1 tsp lemon juice
- 2 tsp extra-virgin olive oil
- ½ cup nonfat buttermilk
- 1 ½ tsp kosher salt
- ⅛ tsp freshly ground black pepper

Directions

Combine all ingredients in a medium bowl and stir well until combined.

Serving Suggestions

Serve with fresh cut vegetables, a fresh leafy green salad, as a sandwich or wrap condiment, or as a dip for grilled meats.

Storage

Keep in the refrigerator in an airtight container for up to two weeks. Stir well before serving.

The Ultimate Mediterranean Chicken and Rice

Peter Schultz

This Mediterranean chicken and rice is a riff on a recipe that Sam Wai shared with us. That recipe was, in turn, inspired by a recipe from The New York Times. The critical ingredients here are Greek sea salt from Crete, extra-virgin olive oil from Mistra Estates, and Hinospice #2, from Hinospices LLC.

Yield ~ 6–8 servings
Total Time ~ 1 hour

Ingredients

- 1 large red onion, chopped
- 3 tbsp minced garlic
- 1 cup celery, chopped
- 1 cup carrots, chopped
- ¼ cup lemon juice
- 2 cans diced tomatoes, with juice
- 2 cans diced green chilis (or jalapeños), with juice
- 1 ⅔ cups rice, washed
- 2 ¾ cups water
- 6 large chicken thighs
- ¼ cup chopped parsley
- Greek sea salt and pepper, to taste
- Mistra Estates extra-virgin olive oil, to taste
- Hinospice #2 spicy, to taste

Directions

1. In a 6-qt Dutch oven, lightly brown onions, celery, and carrots in ¼ cup Mistra Estates EVOO until the onions are golden, about 5+ minutes. Add chopped garlic to the vegetable mix and brown, about

2+ minutes. Add more Mistra Estates EVOO, as necessary.

2. Remove onions, celery, carrots, and garlic to a bowl. To this bowl add ¼ cup lemon juice along with salt, pepper, and Hinospice to taste.
3. Generously rub salt, pepper, and spice on chicken, inside and outside. (Chicken may also be marinated one day in advance with salt, pepper, Hinospice, Mistra Estates EVOO, lemon juice, and ¾ cup of Mateo's Medium [or Hot] Salsa.)
4. Preheat oven to 375°F.
5. Using the same Dutch oven (don't clean), lightly brown chicken thighs on all sides. Add salt, pepper, Mistra Estates EVOO, and Hinospice to taste.
6. Add the onions, celery, carrots, and garlic mixture to the Dutch oven, on top of the chicken. Add the canned tomatoes, peppers, and 2 ¾ water to the Dutch oven, on top of the vegetables. Bring to a low boil. Once boiling, put the Dutch oven into the oven, covered. Bake for 35 minutes.
7. Take the Dutch oven out of the oven. Carefully remove chicken and set to the side. Using a wood spoon, add the rice to the vegetable broth; stir all ingredients thoroughly. Return chicken to the Dutch oven, setting thighs gently ON TOP of the vegetable broth. Salt, pepper, and spice tops of thighs to taste.
8. Return Dutch oven (now containing chicken, broth, and rice) to the oven and bake covered for 30 minutes.
9. Remove and check chicken for doneness. Garnish with chopped parsley.

NOTE

For leftovers, re-fry rice with chopped chicken in 2 tbsp of Mistra Estates EVOO. Glorious.

Fennel A.F.

Sarah Fisher

My fave way to use Mistra Estates!

Yield ~ 4 servings
Prep time ~ 15 minutes

Ingredients

- 2–3 large fennel bulbs, finely shaved
- 1 can garbanzo beans, drained and rinsed
- ½ cup coarsely chopped Italian parsley
- Supremes of one orange (squeeze out the leftover flesh and reserve juice)
- ¼ cup halved Kalamata olives
- 1 tbsp sumac
- ½ tsp ground coriander (best if ground with mortar and pestle, or in spice grinder so as not to make too fine)
- Juice of one lemon (add more to taste)
- Generous drizzling of Mistra Estates EVOO

Directions

1. Combine all ingredient and toss!
2. Serve as a side or add arugula for a heartier dinner salad.

Greek Island Fish Salad

Sam Wai

Purity. Simplicity. Perfection.

Yield ~ 6 servings
Prep Time ~ 20 minutes
Total Time ~ 60 minutes

Ingredients

- 2 thawed mild white fish fillets, about 12 ounces (halibut, cod, pollock, or any other mild white fish)

Poaching Liquid

- 2 cups chicken stock
- 1 cup water
- ¼ cup dry white wine
- 12 whole peppercorns
- 1 parsley sprig
- 1 onion slice

Dressing

- 3 tbsp extra-virgin olive oil
- Juice of 1 lemon
- Lemon zest from ½ lemon (use a microplane for best results)
- 1 chopped spring onion (both white and green parts)
- 2 tsp capers
- ¼ tsp salt
- 2 grinder twists each of white and black pepper

Garnish

- 1 tbsp chopped red onion

- 1 chopped spring onion, green part only
- Dill garnish (fresh, but dry may be substituted)
- Final olive oil drizzle, to serve

Directions

1. Put all the poaching liquid in a small saucepan and bring to a boil for 90 seconds to cook off the alcohol.
2. Put the 2 fish fillets in the poaching liquid and turn the burner down as low as possible. It should be at a bare simmer. Poach the fish to cook through. (It should take no more than 5 minutes, if fully immersed.)
3. Take fish out of the liquid and pat dry. Break fish fillets into large flakes. (Don't overdo it as it will become too fine.)
4. Cover and chill in the fridge.
5. Add all the dressing ingredients and toss lightly to blend. Spread a layer on the flat serving plate, cover and chill until serving. Dish can be prepped in advance and kept cold in the fridge until serving.
6. At service time, put garnish ingredients on top with a final drizzle of olive oil.

Variations

You may add a little chopped cucumber, drained tomatoes, extra lemon juice, olive oil, salt, and pepper to taste. Serve with crisp dry white wine, dry Greek white wine, or Greek retsina.

Rustic Tomato Basil Soup

Julie Garden-Robinson

Tomatoes are known for their high amounts of lycopene, which is a carotenoid pigment that gives tomatoes their red color. Lycopene has been linked to reducing the risk of certain types of cancer and is better absorbed if the tomatoes have been cooked or canned. Enjoy all the flavors of your garden in this delicious soup.

Ingredients

- 2 ½ pounds fresh, ripe tomatoes, halved
- 4 tbsp olive oil
- ½ tbsp salt
- 1 tsp black pepper, plus more to taste
- 2 medium onions, chopped
- 10 garlic cloves, chopped
- 2 - 14 ½-ounce cans fire-roasted tomatoes, with juices
- 3 cups fresh basil leaves, lightly packed
- 2 tsp dried oregano
- 6 cups unsalted vegetable stock
- 1 tsp sugar, depending on sweetness of tomatoes

Directions

1. Preheat oven to 400°F. In a large rimmed sheet pan, combine the fresh tomatoes, 2 tbsp of the olive oil, salt, and pepper. Roast in an even layer for 45 to 60 minutes. While tomatoes are roasting, in a heavy large pot, sauté onions in olive oil for 1 minute. Add garlic and sauté another minute. Add the fire-roasted tomatoes with juices, fresh basil, oregano, and vegetable stock. Stir to combine well.
2. Add your oven-roasted tomatoes (and any liquid that may be on baking sheet) and bring to a low boil. Simmer for 30 minutes uncovered. Use an immersion blender or food processor to puree soup to desired texture. Add 1 tsp of sugar to taste, if needed. Add additional salt and/or black pepper as needed.

Winter Grain Bowl

Cady Ann Rutter

A super fun snack for those colder days on the High Plains!

Yield ~ 2 servings
Prep time ~ 15 minutes
Total time ~ 45 minutes

Ingredients

- 1 ½ cups uncooked brown rice, rinsed
- 2 medium sweet potatoes, peeled and chopped into ½-inch cubes
- 1 - 14.5 ounce can chickpeas, drained, rinsed, and dried
- ½ cup sliced almonds, toasted
- ½ cup dried cranberries, toasted
- 1 pack halloumi cheese, drained and dried
- 2 ounces arugula, or other leafy green of choice
- 5 tbsp extra-virgin olive oil, more to serve

Tahini dressing

- ½ tsp ground cumin
- ½ cup tahini
- Salt
- 3 tbsp lemon juice
- 1 tbsp white wine vinegar
- 2 tbsp extra-virgin olive oil
- ¼ tsp cayenne pepper
- 1 clove minced fresh garlic, or ¼ tsp garlic power
- Dash of smoked paprika
- 2–4 tbsp ice water

To serve: Hot honey, extra-virgin olive oil

DIRECTIONS

1. Preheat oven to 425°F.
2. Cook brown rice according to package instructions. Set aside, covered.
3. Meanwhile, toss the sweet potatoes and chickpeas in 3 tbsp of olive oil and arrange on a parchment-lined baking sheet. Season with sea salt and black pepper to taste.
4. Roast for 25–30 minutes, or until the sweet potatoes are fork tender.
5. Prepare the tahini dressing by whisking together the cumin, tahini, a pinch of salt, lemon juice, white wine vinegar, olive oil, cayenne, paprika, garlic, and 2 tbsp of the ice water in a medium bowl. Add additional ice water by the teaspoon until a drizzling consistency is reached. Set aside.
6. Cut the halloumi cheese into ½-inch planks and cook in 1 tbsp of olive oil in a medium-sized skillet over medium heat until golden, approximately 6–8 minutes on each side. Set aside.
7. To now empty skillet, add arugula and cook on medium low until soft and wilted.
8. Assemble bowls with rice, sweet potatoes, chickpeas, almonds, cranberries, arugula, and halloumi.
9. Drizzle tahini dressing, hot honey, and additional olive oil over prepared bowls and serve.

APPENDIX B
HOW DO YOU BUY THE VERY BEST EXTRA VIRGIN OLIVE OIL?

PETER SCHULTZ, PHD

In 2011, Tom Mueller published his book *Extra Virginity. The Sublime and Scandalous World of Olive Oil.* This book followed closely on the heels of a (now infamous!) 2010 report on "extra-virgin olive oil" by scholars from the UC Davis Olive Oil Center at the Robert Mondavi Institute for Wine and Food Science and the University of California, Davis. The conclusion of these important publications was identical: The world of olive oil is rife with inaccuracies, half-truths, and fraud.

The UC Davis study concludes:

> Of the five top-selling imported "extra-virgin" olive oil brands in the United States, 73 percent of the samples *failed* the IOC sensory standards for extra-virgin olive oils analyzed by two IOC-accredited sensory panels. The failure rate ranged from a high of 94 percent to a low of 56 percent depending on the brand and the panel. None of the Australian and Californian samples failed both sensory panels, while 11 percent of the top-selling premium Italian brand samples failed the two panels. Sensory defects are indicators that these samples are oxidized, of poor quality, and/or adulterated with cheaper refined oils.

In the last decade or so, this research has been substantiated time and time again, leaving all of us who love the Mediterranean diet with a serious question: *How do you buy the very* best *extra-virgin olive oil?*

The good news is that this is a very easy question to answer!

Here's a fast, fun, fact-based checklist of three key criteria that you can use to find and buy the highest quality extra-virgin olive oil.

1. Your extra-virgin olive oil should always come in ceramic, in dark glass, or in a stainless-steel tin; it should never be stored a clear bottle—and it should never come in plastic.
Photons—light—degrade the quality of extra-virgin olive oil. Indeed, any exposure to light can cause a substantial loss of key antioxidants, especially tocopherols, and an increase in rancidity compared to oil stored in the dark. For this reason, an opaque or dark container is a must.

A glass or steel container is also very important. In 2018, Maryam Hooshyari and her colleagues at the Università degli Studi di Genova conducted a series of studies that showed that olive oil stored in plastic bottles or bags undergo far more rapid oxidation due to the permeability of PET (polyethylene terephthalate) plastic. Plastics also contains BPA (bisphenol A). BPA is an industrial chemical that has been used to make popular plastics and resins since the 1960s. Polycarbonate plastics are often used in containers that store food and beverages, such as water bottles. They may also be used in other consumer goods. Epoxy resins are used to coat the inside of metal products, such as food cans, bottle tops, and water supply lines. Research has shown that BPA can seep into food or beverages from containers that are made with BPA. Exposure to BPA is a concern because of possible health effects on the brain and prostate glands of fetuses, infants, and children. It can also affect children's behavior. Additional research suggests a possible link between BPA and increased blood pressure. Ceramic, glass, or steel are the best ways to go.

2. Your extra-virgin olive oil's label should always display a harvest and/or season date and a documented acidity level.
Research has shown that it takes next to nothing for an unscrupulous manufacturer to label an oil "cold-pressed" or "extra-virgin." Also, even olive oil that is technically "extra-virgin" can spoil, especially when it's brought into the United States in multi-ton bulk orders and stored for long periods of time in shipping containers, warehouses, or grocery stores. Acidity level is also a key indicator of quality and should always be shown on the label.

The two best ways to address this concern are to be sure that (1) the label of your extra-virgin olive oil is marked with a *harvest date* and (2) the label of your extra-virgin olive oil is marked with a *documented level of acidity*.

With regards to date, it's important to remember that olive oil is a seasonal product. In the northern hemisphere, the olive harvest usually takes between October and January. Here in the US, the very freshest olive oil from a harvest year will arrive in the late spring and summer. While it can last three to four years when stored in a cool, dry place, an olive oil's very best flavor will manifest within two years of the harvest date. (Truly fresh extra-virgin olive oil is almost a miracle to taste; once you have it, it's almost impossible to go back.) Be sure that when you're looking at your oil's harvest date that it's not more than two years old.

With regards to acidity, less is always more. The lower acidity, the better. In order to technically qualify as "extra-virgin olive oil," an oil must have an acidity of less than 0.8 percent. Anything below this number is a good product. Extra-virgin olive oils with a range of 0–0.6 percent acidity are some of the very best in the world. Tasting an early pressing of green olives at 0.0 percent acidity can be life-changing.

3. Your extra-virgin olive oil should always come from a single farm or a regional co-op. In other words, know who grows and harvests your food.

The vast majority of extra-virgin olive oil in the supermarket is comprised of industrial blends derived from multiple production sites and even multiple countries. The goals of these producers are volume and economies of scale. These goals are entirely fine, of course, but they're incompatible with elite quality. If you want the very best extra-virgin olive oil in the world, then buy from a family farm or a regional co-op. These outfits usually take great care of their land, guarantee the freshest products in the world, and take enormous pride in the quality of their oil. Even more important, discovering high-quality farms is a blast and building relationships with the people who grow and make what you eat will always have rewards that go far beyond mere sustenance. It's quite easy to find high-quality olive oil of this sort. The internet offers a vast range of local growers and, if you're up in the High Plains of the American Midwest, you can always sign up for our annual order of Mistra Estates olive oil at www.peterschultzimporter.com!

Select Bibliography

Chapter One
A Brief History of the Siesta

Ji, X., J. Li, and J. Liu. "The Relationship Between Midday Napping and Neurocognitive Function in Early Adolescents." *Behavioral Sleep Medicine* 17, no. 5 (2019): 537–51.

Boukhris, O., K. Trabelsi, D. W. Hill, et al. "Physiological Response and Physical Performance after 40 Min and 90 Min Daytime Nap Opportunities." *Research in Sports Medicine* 31, no. 6 (2023): 881–94.

Burazeri, G., J. Gofin, and J. D. Kark. "Siesta and Mortality in a Mediterranean Population: A Community Study in Jerusalem." *Sleep* 26, no. 5 (2003): 578–84.

Cai, M., Y. Huang, X. Sun, Y. He, and C. Sun. "Siesta Is Associated with Reduced Systolic Blood Pressure Level and Decreased Prevalence of Hypertension in Older Adults." *Journal of Human Hypertension* 30 (2016):216–18.

Häusler, N., J. Haba-Rubio, R. Heinzer, and P. Marques-Vidal. "Association of Napping with Incident Cardiovascular Events in a Prospective Cohort Study." *Heart* 105, no.23 (2019): 1793–798.

Kang, H., X. Feng, B. Zhang, et al. "The Siesta Habit is Associated with a Decreased Risk of Rupture of Intracranial Aneurysms." *Frontiers in Neurology* 8 (2017): 451.

Kreouzi, M., N. Theodorakis, and C. Constantinou. "Lessons Learned from Blue Zones, Lifestyle Medicine Pillars and Beyond: An Update on the Contributions of Behavior and Genetics to Wellbeing and Longevity." *American Journal of Lifestyle Medicine* 18, no. 6 (2024): 750–65.

Kushkestani, M., M. Moghadassi, and L. Sidossis. "Mediterranean Lifestyle: More than a Diet, a Way of Living (and Thriving)." *Endocrine, Metabolic & Immune Disorders-Drug Targets* 24, no. 15 (2024): 1785–93.

Lin, L., J. Huang, Z. Liu, P. Chen, and C. Huang. "Associations of Siesta and Total Sleep Duration with Hypertension or Cardiovascular Diseases in Middle-Aged and Older Adults." *Clinical Cardiology* 46, no. 2 (2023): 159–70.

Lou, S., S. Hu, Y. Chen, et al. "Benefits of Napping Habits in Healthy Adults: Maintaining Alerting Performance and Cortisol Levels Change within 90 Min of Habitual Napping Time." *Sleep Medicine* 119 (2024): 214–21.

Luo, Z., and S. Inoué. "A Short Daytime Nap Modulates Levels of Emotions Objectively Evaluated by the Emotion Spectrum Analysis Method." *Psychiatry and Clinical Neurosciences* 54, no. 2 (2000): 207–212.

Mangat, S., and A. Razzaq Carmichael. "The Science of Midday Napping and Islam." *The Review of Religions*, August 23, 2023.

Mohammad, Y. "Siesta and Risk for Ischemic Stroke: Results from a Case-Control Study." *Medicina* 56, no. 5 (2020): 222.

Murphy, P. J., and S. S. Campbell. "Therapeutic Benefits of Napping in the Elderly." In *Principles and Practice of Geriatric Sleep Medicine*, edited by S. R. Pandi-Perumal, Jaime M. Monti, and Andrew A. Monjan, 413–22. Cambridge University Press, 2009.

Paraskakis, E., M. Hitas, T. Ntouros, M. Ntokos, A. Hatzimichail, and M. Kalmanti. "Siesta and Sleep Habits of Adolescents in Greece." *Pediatrics* 121, no. Supplement_2 (2008): S90.

Pérez, A. Fernández-Cruz, and R. Gabriel Sánchez. "El reloj biológico, la hora de la cena y la siesta en España. Su impacto en la longevidad." *Anales de la Real Academia Nacional de Medicina* 136, no. 2 (2019): 201.

Sidossis, L. S., R. Lawson, E. Aprilakis, et al. "Defining the Traditional Mediterranean Lifestyle: Joint International Consensus Statement." *Lifestyle Medicine* 5, no. 4 (2024): e115.

Stefanadis, C. I. "Unveiling the Secrets of Longevity: The Ikaria Study." *Hellenic Journal of Cardiology* 52, no. 5 (2011): 479–80.

Trichopoulos, D., A. Tzonou, C. Christopoulos, S. Havatzoglou, and A.Trichopoulou. "Siesta and Risk of Coronary Heart Disease." *Stress Medicine* 4, no. 3 (1988): 143–8.

Vgontzas, A. N., S. Pejovic, E. Zoumakis, et al. "Daytime Napping after a Night of Sleep Loss Decreases Sleepiness, Improves Performance, and Causes Beneficial Changes in Cortisol and Interleukin-6 Secretion." *American Journal of Physiology-Endocrinology and Metabolism* 292, no. 1 (2007): E253–E261.

Chapter Five
The Mediterranean See: Eyes, Diet, and Vision

Agrón, E., et al. "Adherence to a Mediterranean Diet and Geographic Atrophy Enlargement Rate: Age-Related Eye Disease Study 2 Report 29." *Ophthalmology Retina* 6, no. 9 (2022): 762–70.

Alanazi, S. A., et al. "Effects of Short-Term Oral Vitamin A Supplementation on the Ocular Tear Film in Patients with Dry Eye." *Clinical Ophthalmology* 13 (2019): 599–604.

American Academy of Ophthalmology. "Age-Related Macular Degeneration Preferred Practice Pattern." https://www.aao.org/education/preferred-practice-pattern/age-related-macular-degeneration-ppp.

Barbouti, A., and V. Goulas. "Dietary Antioxidants in the Mediterranean Diet." *Antioxidants* 10, no. 8 (2021): 1213.

Bryl, A., et al. "A Mediterranean Diet May Be Protective in the Development of Diabetic Retinopathy." *International Journal of Molecular Sciences* 24, no. 13 (2023): 11145.

Dogru, M., et al. "Potential Role of Oxidative Stress in Ocular Surface Inflammation and Dry Eye Disease." *Investigative Ophthalmology & Visual Science* 59, no. 14 (2018): DES163–DES68.

Favero, G., et al. "Evidence of Polyphenols Efficacy against Dry Eye Disease." *Antioxidants* 10, no. 2 (2021): 190.

Gorzynik-Debicka, M., et al. "Potential Health Benefits of Olive Oil and Plant Polyphenols." *International Journal of Molecular Sciences* 19, no. 3 (2018): 686.

Hogg, R. E., et al. "Mediterranean Diet Score and Its Association with Age-Related Macular Degeneration: The European Eye Study." *Ophthalmology* 124, no. 1 (2017): 82–89.

Latib, F. (Ratib), et al. "The Use of Vitamin E in Ocular Health: Bridging Omics Approaches with Tocopheral and Tocotrienol in the Management of Glaucoma." *Food Chemistry: Molecular Sciences* 9 (2024): 100224.

Lin, P., et al. "A Review of the Role of the Intestinal Microbiota in Age-Related Macular Degeneration." *Journal of Clinical Medicine* 10, no. 10 (2021): 2072.

Macsai, M. S. "The Role of Omega-3 Dietary Supplementation in Blepharitis and Meibomian Gland Dysfunction (An AOS Thesis)." *Transactions of American Ophthalmological Society* 106 (2008): 336–56.

Molina-Leyva, I., et al. "Effectiveness of Mediterranean Diet Implementation in Dry Eye Parameters: A Study of PREDIMED-PLUS Trial." *Nutrients* 12, no. 5 (2020): 1289.

Mrowicka, M., et al. "Lutein and Zeaxanthin and Their Roles in Age-Related Macular Degeneration-Neurodegenerative Disease." *Nutrients* 14, no. 4 (2022): 827.

Schwab, I. R. *Evolution's Witness: How Eyes Evolved*. Oxford University Press, 2012.

Chapter Six
The Mediterranean Table: A Prescription for Cancer Prevention and Survivorship

Buettner, D., and S. Skemp. "Blue Zones: Lessons from the world's longest-lived." *American Journal of Lifestyle Medicine* 10, no. 5 (2016): 318–21.

Christakis, N. A., and J. H. Fowler. "The spread of obesity in a large social network over 32 years." *New England Journal of Medicine* 357, no. 4 (2007): 370–9.

Colditz, G. A., and K. Y. Wolin. "Preventable cancer cases in the U.S.: The role of lifestyle changes." *Science Translational Medicine* 4, no. 127 (2012): 127rv4.

De Filippis, F., N. Pellegrini, L. Vannini, et al. "High-level adherence to a Mediterranean diet beneficially impacts the gut microbiome and associated metabolome." *Gut* 69, no. 6 (2020): 1218–28.

Donohoe, D. R., L. B. Collins, A. Wali, et al. "The Warburg effect dictates the mechanism of butyrate-mediated histone acetylation and cell proliferation." *Molecular Cell* 48, no. 4 (2012): 612–26. https://doi.org/10.1016/j.molcel.2012.08.033.

Esposito, K., et al. "Effect of a Mediterranean-style diet on endothelial dysfunction and markers of vascular inflammation in the metabolic syndrome: A randomized trial." *JAMA* 289, no. 14 (2003): 1799–1804.

Estruch, R., et al. "Effects of a Mediterranean-style diet on weight loss and risk factors associated with metabolic syndrome: Results of a randomized trial." *Annals of Internal Medicine* 152, no. 11 (2010): 667–75.

Estruch, R., E. Ros, J. Salas-Salvadó, et al. "Primary Prevention of Cardiovascular Disease with a Mediterranean Diet Supplemented with Extra-Virgin Olive Oil or Nuts." *The New England Journal of Medicine* 372, no. 14 (2015): 1378–88. https://doi.org/10.1056/NEJMoa1800389.

Goodwin, P. J., et al. "The Effect of Group Psychosocial Support on Survival in Metastatic Breast Cancer." *New England Journal of Medicine* 345, no. 24 (2001): 1719–26.

Kroenke, C. H., et al. "Social Networks, Social Support, and Survival after Breast Cancer Diagnosis." *Journal of Clinical Oncology* 24, no. 7 (2006): 1105–11.

Kroenke, C. H., T. T. Fung, F. B. Hu, et al. "Dietary Patterns and Survival after Breast Cancer Diagnosis." *JNCI: Journal of the National Cancer Institute* 97, no. 7 (2005): 517–24. https://doi.org/10.1200/JCO.2005.02.0198.

Lampe, J. W., and J. L. Chang. "Interindividual Differences in Phytochemical Metabolism and Disposition." *Seminars in Cancer Biology* 17, no. 5 (2007): 368–74. https://doi.org/10.1016/j.semcancer.2007.05.003.

Murphy, N., T. Norat, P. Ferrari, et al. "Dietary Fiber Intake and Risk of Colorectal Cancer in the European Prospective Investigation into Cancer and Nutrition (EPIC) Study." *JNCI: Journal of the National Cancer Institute* 111, no. 6 (2019): 543–53.

Pinquart, M., and P. R. Duberstein. "Associations of Social Networks with Cancer Mortality: A Meta-Analysis." *Critical Reviews in Oncology/Hematology* 75, no. 2 (2010): 122–37.

Rosignoli, P., R. Fuccelli, R. Fabiani, et al. "Hydroxytyrosol, a Natural Antioxidant from Olive Oil, Prevents DNA Damage and Induces Apoptosis in Colon Cancer Cells." *Nutritional Cancer* 65, no. 5 (2013): 793–8.

Schwingshackl, L., G. Hoffmann, A. M. Lampousi, et al. "Food Groups and Risk of Colorectal Cancer." *International Journal of Cancer* 142, no. 9 (2017): 1748–58. https://doi.org/10.1002/ijc.31198.

Shivappa, N., S. E. Steck, T. G. Hurley, et al. "The Inflammatory Potential of the Mediterranean Diet Score Is Associated with Colorectal Cancer Risk in a Large Italian Case-Control Study." *Nutrients* 10, no. 5 (2018): 634.

Sotos-Prieto, M., et al. "Association of Changes in Diet Quality with Total and Cause-Specific Mortality." *New England Journal of Medicine* 373, no. 9 (2015): 1–10.

Spiegel, D., et al. "Effect of Psychosocial Treatment on Survival of Patients with Metastatic Breast Cancer." *The Lancet* 334, no. 8668 (1989): 888–91.

Toledo, E., J. Salas-Salvadó, C. Donat-Vargas, et al. "Mediterranean Diet and Invasive Breast Cancer Risk among Women at High Cardiovascular Risk in the PREDIMED Trial: A Randomized Clinical Trial." *JAMA Internal Medicine* 175, no. 11 (2015): 1752–60. https://doi.org/10.1001/jamainternmed.2015.4838.

Tresserra-Rimbau, A., et al. "Adherence to a Mediterranean Diet and Excessive Weight among Spanish University Graduates: The SUN Project." *British Journal of Nutrition* 119, no. 11 (2018): 1201–10.

Uchino, B. N. "Social Support and Health: A Review of Physiological Processes Potentially Underlying Links to Disease Outcomes." *Journal of Behavioral Medicine* 29, no. 4 (2006): 377–87.

Yang, H. C., et al. "Social Support, Emotion Regulation, and Depression in Breast Cancer Patients: A Longitudinal Analysis." *Journal of Behavioral Medicine* 33, no. 1 (2010): 48–57.

Yannakoulia, M., et al. "Mediterranean Diet and Obesity: Current Evidence." *Nutrition Reviews* 66, no. 2 (2008): 39–46.

Chapter Seven
Socrates Visits the Doctor: The Mediterranean Diet and Quality of Life

Fransen, H. P., J. W. Beulens, A. M. May, et al. "Dietary Patterns in Relation to Quality-Adjusted Life Years in the EPIC-NL Cohort." *Preventive Medicine* 77 (2015): 119–24. https://doi.org/10.1016/j.ypmed.2015.05.014.

Augustovski, F., L. D. Colantonio, J. Galante, et al. "Measuring the Benefits of Healthcare: DALYs and QALYs - Does the Choice of Measure Matter? A Case Study of Two Preventive Interventions." *International Journal of Health Policy and Management* 7, no. 2 (2018): 120–36. https://doi.org/10.15171/ijhpm.2017.47.

May, A. M., E. A. Struijk, H. P. Fransen, et al. "The Impact of a Healthy Lifestyle on Disability-Adjusted Life Years: A Prospective Cohort Study." *BMC Medicine* 13, no. 39 (2015). https://doi.org/10.1186/s12916-015-0287-6.

Martinez-Gonzalez, M. A., and N. Martin-Calvo. "Mediterranean Diet and Life Expectancy; Beyond Olive Oil, Fruits, and Vegetables." *Current Opinion in Clinical Nutrition and Metabolic Care* 19, no. 6 (2016): 401–407. https://doi.org/10.1097/MCO.0000000000000316.

Veronese, N., B. Stubbs, M. Noale, M. Solmi, C. Luchini, and S. Maggi. "Adherence to the Mediterranean Diet Is Associated with Better Quality of Life: Data from the Osteoarthritis Initiative." *The American Journal of Clinical Nutrition* 104, no. 5 (2016): 1403–9. https://doi.org/10.3945/ajcn.116.136390.

Cabrera-Suárez, B. M., F. Lahortiga-Ramos, C. Sayon-Orea, et al. "Effect of a Dietary Intervention Based on the Mediterranean Diet on the Quality of Life of Patients Recovered from Depression: Analysis of the PREDIDEP Randomized Trial." *Experimental Gerontology* 175 (2023): 112149. https://doi.org/10.1016/j.exger.2023.112149.

Godos, J., G. Grosso, R. Ferri, et al. "Mediterranean Diet, Mental Health, Cognitive Status, Quality of Life, and Successful Aging in Southern Italian Older Adults." *Experimental Gerontology* 175 (2023): 112143. https://doi.org/10.1016/j.exger.2023.112143.

Schwarzinger, M., and C. Dufouil. "Forecasting the Prevalence of Dementia." Lancet Public Health 7, no. 2 (2022): e94–e95. https://doi.org/10.1016/S2468-2667(21)00277-2.

Made in the USA
Monee, IL
05 November 2026

67387534R00069